HUMAN ECOLOGY IN SPACE FLIGHT III

Proceedings of the Third International Interdisciplinary Conference

Edited by
DORIS HOWES CALLOWAY

This Conference was sponsored by the Office of Naval Research and the National Aeronautics and Space Administration. The Conference was held at Princeton, New Jersey from October 10 to 13, 1965.

PUBLISHED BY:
THE NEW YORK ACADEMY OF SCIENCES
INTERDISCIPLINARY COMMUNICATIONS PROGRAM
NEW YORK, NEW YORK

PARTICIPANTS

Third Conference on Human Ecology in Space Flight

WALLACE O. FENN, *Chairman*
Department of Physiology
University of Rochester School of Medicine and Dentistry
Rochester, New York

DORIS HOWES CALLOWAY, *Editor*
Department of Nutritional Sciences, University of California
Berkeley, California

WALTER E. ARNOLDI
Hamilton Standard, Division of United Aircraft Corp.
Windsor Locks, Connecticut

RICHARD H. BARNES
Graduate School of Nutrition, Cornell University
Ithaca, New York

JOHN R. BROBECK
Department of Physiology
University of Pennsylvania School of Medicine
Philadelphia, Pennsylvania

ALLAN H. BROWN
Department of Biology, University of Pennsylvania
Philadelphia, Pennsylvania

ALAN N. EPSTEIN
Department of Biology, University of Pennsylvania
Philadelphia, Pennsylvania

BENGT E. GUSTAFSSON
Department of Germfree Research, Karolinska Institute
Stockholm, Sweden

FRANKLIN W. HEGGENESS
Department of Physiology
University of Rochester School of Medicine and Dentistry
Rochester, New York

DALE W. JENKINS
Bioscience Programs, Office of Space Science and Applications
National Aeronautics and Space Administration
Washington, District of Columbia

ROBERT W. KRAUSS
Department of Botany, University of Maryland
College Park, Maryland

ROBERT B. LIVINGSTON
Department of Neurosciences
University of California, San Diego, School of Medicine
La Jolla, California

JEAN MAYER
Department of Nutrition, Harvard University School of Public Health
Boston, Massachusetts

D. A. A. MOSSEL
Central Institute for Nutrition and Food Research, TNO
Zeist, The Netherlands

H. N. MUNRO
Department of Biochemistry, University of Glasgow
Glasgow, Scotland

MORRIS POLLARD
Department of Biology, University of Notre Dame
Notre Dame, Indiana

HERMANN RAHN
Department of Physiology, State University of New York at Buffalo
Buffalo, New York

ORR E. REYNOLDS
Bioscience Programs, Office of Space Science and Applications
National Aeronautics and Space Administration
Washington, District of Columbia

DAVID R. SCHWARZ
Schwarz BioResearch, Inc.
Orangeburg, New York

Klaus Schwarz
Department of Biological Chemistry
University of California School of Medicine
Los Angeles, California

B. S. Schweigert
Department of Food Science, Michigan State University
East Lansing, Michigan

A. L. Tappel
Department of Food Science and Technology, University of California
Davis, California

Calvin H. Ward
Environmental Systems Branch, USAF School of Aerospace Medicine
Brooks Air Force Base, Texas

THE NEW YORK ACADEMY OF SCIENCES

INTERDISCIPLINARY COMMUNICATIONS PROGRAM

Dr. Frank Fremont-Smith, *Director*

Mrs. Elizabeth Purcell
Miss Patricia Gordon

TABLE OF CONTENTS

Introductory remarks
F. Fremont-Smith 9

I. Introduction to the problems posed to the Conference 11
Discussion leader:
Wallace O. Fenn

II. The macronutrients 28
Discussion leader:
Doris Howes Calloway

III. The micronutrients 54
Discussion leader:
Klaus Schwarz

IV. Appetite, satiety and food acceptance 92
Discussion leaders:
John R. Brobeck and Frank W. Heggenness

V. Intestinal microflora and germfree life 119
Discussion leader:
Bengt E. Gustafsson

VI. Regenerative systems reexamined 160
Discussion leader:
Dale Jenkins

VII. Last words 204
Discussion leaders:
Wallace O. Fenn and H. N. Munro

References 232

Index 237

INTRODUCTORY REMARKS

The Conference which this publication attempts faithfully to report had as its purpose a multidiscipline discussion in depth of topics that are increasingly challenging the attention of scientists in many fields. Perhaps, then, it is not inappropriate that I present at the outset here a few of my basic assumptions. The major one is that nature is all of one piece. The second one is that as we get more information, more data flowing in at an increasingly rapid rate, we are faced with the realization that the area of ignorance is much larger than we thought. Wouldn't you agree with me that the half-life of facts is getting shorter and shorter?

There is almost no systematic effort made to provide for interdiscipline communication, nor multidiscipline discussion. If what I am saying is true about the rate of inflow of new information, if we have reached the point—and I think we have—where no one ever again can claim that he is up-to-date even in the narrowest area of science, then we must accept the fact that never again can anyone fool himself into feeling he knows the last word in any science, no matter how narrow. What we have to do is accept a limitation in having only a relative sample of what is going on in any particular area; and if we wish to participate in the breakthroughs or to understand them when other people make them, we must also have a relative sample of the data from disciplines related to our area of special concern. At the present time there is little systematic effort to make this possible. This is what we are about, and we think it terribly important, because we believe that this is the essence of science.

We believe that the standard publications really falsify science because they give a logical progression; but this was not the way the research was done. The research went here and there, and started over here again with another idea, and finally it ended up here; but the man who started this research left a little flag where he began and now he draws the line back to that little flag and this is what he publishes—a simple, straight, logical process.

This is not the way it happened. It is to some degree a false picture of science. It fools us and it fools our students and discourages really imaginative students from attempting anything as dull as a purely logical process. Logic is very important, but it is not the creative aspect.

We used to be brought up with the idea that one observes phenomena and then takes a second step and interprets it, but I think there is a great deal of evidence from many sides to show that this is not the case, really—that what we do is to build an interpretation directly into the initial observation. Therefore, all observations are really interpretations based on observations in our own past. It is impossible for us to be a *tabula rasa;* we always see anything we perceive in the light of something in our past, so we are trailing clouds, not of glory, but of the past as we approach each new phenomenon. This means that all of us put our special coloring of our own past experience on what we see or hear or observe, and, therefore, all of us put, to some degree, a falseness, a distortion upon our observations. It is very important that we become aware of this and, instead of denying it, take account of it and do such things as can be done to counterbalance it.

These distorting lenses and deaf spots and blind spots that we carry around with us, however, are not absolutely fixed objects. You can see the distorting lenses bending in the presence of hostility or anxiety, or you can see the lenses flattening out—people may even take them off and put them down on the table—if you can set up the appropriate atmosphere (and we hope we have). The blind spots will disappear, the deaf spots will shrink, and you will see each other and suddenly begin to understand each other.

FRANK FREMONT-SMITH, DIRECTOR
Interdisciplinary Communications Program
The New York Academy of Sciences
New York, New York

I. INTRODUCTION TO THE PROBLEMS POSED TO THE CONFERENCE

Discussion Leader:

WALLACE O. FENN
Department of Physiology
University of Rochester
School of Medicine and Dentistry
Rochester, New York

FENN: I would like to begin by making one comment on the purpose of this Conference.

One of the obligations of NASA is to exploit the space age and space travel for the advancement of science, making sure that we do not miss any experiments that might be done in space. Space makes natural experiments for us, just as disease does, and presents an opportunity to advance science, and part of the objective, therefore, of such a Conference as this is to explore broadly the implications of space and of possible things that might happen, the possible experiments that might be done for us by space travel, and to make sure that we get the greatest good out of it.

FREMONT-SMITH: Unfortunately, our scientific community seems much more willing to listen to a series of speeches, or to make a series of speeches, and to limit its communication effort to listening to or objecting to the idea of an individual; but, really, does our scientific community provide the setting in which an idea may be examined and reexamined by others who approach the problem from a different point of view? This is what we hope to do. We think it is unusual.

MAYER: Dr. Fremont-Smith, may I make a comment on the last (Nutrition-in-Space) Conference and this one? I was at the last Conference, as a number of people here were. I did not like it at all.

FREMONT-SMITH: You mean the last Conference here?

MAYER: No, the (NASA) Conference in Tampa, Florida (in April, 1964).[1] The reason I did not like it is that what essentially we were dealing with, was a series of engineering problems, in terms of the practical aspects of space exploration.

Now, those engineering problems in turn are dependent for their solution on the solution of scientific problems which we may or may not have the answers to, or, for that matter, problems of which we were not aware until the engineering problems arose.

At the same time what we were being asked to do at Tampa was essentially to contribute answers when the questions had not been defined, and I felt intensely frustrated throughout the whole Conference, because practically everybody gave the little speech he would have given under any circumstances, and hoped vaguely that it had something to do with the problems of NASA. At no time did the problems of NASA really get properly explained to us, so that we could give intelligent answers.

Now, I hope that if the purpose of this Conference is to provide useful guidance to the people who are going to deal with the engineering, practical problems at NASA, they are going to be a little bit more specific as to what they think at present the conditions are under which the people are going to go into space as regards physiology, nutrition, and so on. Otherwise, I think we will again have this feeling of unreality, of discussing what we are interested in in a sort of very vague context of minimum ecological systems for man in space.

FREMONT-SMITH: I think we suffered somewhat from the same difficulty in the last two Conferences held by this group, and I wonder whether either Dr. Reynolds or Dr. Jenkins would wish to make a comment now or wish to volunteer whether it is possible to answer the questions that have been raised, or whether the fact is that we have to struggle with situations which are at the moment unknown, or partly unknown, and try to anticipate by exchange of ideas some of the developments that either will be made or need to be made. I suspect the situation is changing and that perhaps we have to discuss where we have stood, where we are standing, and where we hope to stand.

REYNOLDS: The way I, at least, have looked on the utility of this kind of a Conference is not to try to provide concrete answers to engineering or practical problems that we have, but to find ways of illuminating the science underlying the field, so as to prompt further research on the science, not to try to anticipate the engineering problems. It seems to me that it is particularly applicable in this case, because we really do not know what the engineering problems are going to be or in what time period they are going to arrive.

FENN: I think you are asking for answers where you have not defined the question. Perhaps you are asking Dr. Reynolds and Dr. Jenkins to define the question more accurately in part, and I hope they will do that, and give us as much answer as they can.

FREMONT-SMITH: Finally, Dr. Fenn gave me a chance to tell a favorite story that some of you have already heard.

This takes me to Gertrude Stein's deathbed scene. Of course, Alice Toklas was there, and Gertrude was very restless and unhappy and miserable, and Alice was trying to comfort her and quiet her, and she wouldn't be quieted. She kept saying, "Alice, what is the answer? What is the answer?"

And Alice tried to quiet her down, but she wouldn't be. "What is the answer?" Alice finally felt that the only thing she could do was to tell Gertrude the truth, even at this last moment of her life, and she said, "Gertrude, there is no answer."

"If no answer, then what is the question?"

K. SCHWARZ: To give you a very simple example, I for one did not even know what the gas phase is in the capsule as it stands now, and I got on the telephone and asked Dr. Calloway, and she said: So far, it's oxygen.

These simple facts are missing to some of us, and it would be very helpful if you would just outline the physiological situation as it stands now, and what is known specifically about dangerous or damaging events which may have happened so far.

REYNOLDS: Ecological systems of the types that we are talking about here are relevant to extended lunar or interplanetary flights—missions for which there are no concrete engineering plans. We have not established the size of the groups of people that we are going to carry. We don't know exactly what boosters will be involved, and therefore what the time scales are.

All we know is that we are probably going to be put in the position of having to provide for a man's total requirements for extended periods of time under conditions such as we have never encountered before, and it seems to me this constitutes a good reason for a thoroughly better understanding of what the interrelations between man and his environment are, which we have not had in the past.

MAYER: This certainly calls for a greater knowledge, but we are talking about a three-day Conference in which we are not going to review all of biology, all of nutrition, all of physiology, and therefore it seems to me that some working models would give us a least some framework.

The trip to Mars at one time was going to take a year, and a year to come back, and if this is the time span we anticipate, it seems to me it would be useful to talk about it, so that we would have some sort of framework, rather than go all over science in three days.

REYNOLDS: With the current range of energy capability in boosters, the first time that it looks practical to send a man to Mars for a stay, not just an orbit and return, would be about twenty years from now; 1984 would be the date, when Mars has its closest opposition after the forthcoming 1971 opposition. If you have a landing, the chances are that, again assuming present booster capabilities, it would take eight months to get there, almost two years of residence on the surface, and eights months to return.

The problem with that is that this assumes no major technical advances in launch vehicles, and since that is twenty years off, and since we said ten years ago that to talk about trying to support men in space was silly, I think it would be not very wise to assume there are not going to be any changes in the technology.

That is one of the reasons that I do not think it is too valuable to try to pin this kind of Conference to studies based on present technological capabilities. I think we would be a lot better off to improve the state of science, so that we can use it appropriately as the technology advances.

FREMONT-SMITH: In other words, to exchange basic ideas about the different aspects of science that contribute to the problem, bearing in mind that we are concerned with the space problem, which will have many facets and many changing facets, but not to hitch our wagon to one particular star.

I would like to quote a radio statement that was made last night, quoting Mr. Webb.

I may not have it quite right, but I am sure I have essentially what the radio man said that Mr. Webb said: With respect to the space problem and the man-machine interrelationship that the machines were just absolutely fine. There was no problem at all; they were really working splendidly, but that the man, the astronaut, just turned out to be a little more human than could have been, or had been anticipated, and that this was the problem that was facing NASA.

My own view of the man-machine interrelationship is that it has been too unilateral, in the sense that the engineers have set things up—excellent things, in many cases, and then man has been forced into them, and the machine could not be much changed, because it had already been set and the blueprints had been arranged for, and man had to fit in there—whatever the results.

Now, I think that we have not had man-knowledgeable people working hand-in-glove with the engineers, as far as I know, while the engineers are making their original plans. It seems to me that this is an essential feature for the future, so that we do not set up engineering problems to which man cannot or cannot without serious loss or danger adapt himself. It seems to me it has got to be an interadaptation between machine and man, in which the machine must adapt as well as the man, and then we get a confluence which will work.

I may be speaking out of my ignorance, which I usually do. It may be that this has been going on, but I have not been able to catch any clue that it really was going on in any genuine sense, and that any of the people who were deeply knowledgeable about man's capacities and human physiology were really involved in the early planning when crystallization of the machine orientation took place.

MAYER: The thing that concerns me is that, while there have been a number of conferences on ecological factors in space, all of which have had extraordinarily vague terms of reference, the immediate data that we could get out of the experiments that are going on now are not very good biologically, and we have just been told that the results really are very vague and that the medical aspects have taken second or tenth place to the engineering aspects.

Now, I think that unless and until there is some point of concrete union between the people who are doing the work at NASA and people such as ourselves, that what we are doing is journalism and science fiction, and we are not really being very useful to the people who are in space, nor are the people who are in space, I think, privy to what good advice they might conceivably get if we were working under somewhat more specific conditions.

ARNOLDI: The question of fixing a target of some sort of mission duration comes back to the question of what developments there will be in propulsion technology, but I am not at all sure that fixing a target is necessary here, or even desirable.

In the first place, because of the uncertainties in propulsion technology it is quite possible that five years or 10 years or 15 years from now we will have continuous propulsion, say, at a tenth of gravity, or something like that and the Mars trip will be two weeks. That would be analogous to the Apollo trip to the moon.

So let us go back to the Apollo mission as an example. If the Apollo mission currently is—talking loosely about all possible planned Apollo missions—of a two weeks to a month order of magnitude time duration, let us assume that such a mission has been successful; that the equipment works; that the people survive. The next question is: how long can somebody stay on the moon?

From an engineering point of view all the equipment that he uses on a short stay can be stretched or modified or replaced to extend the stay to whatever extent is desirable. However, this Conference, I think, is concerned with: What are the human and physiological limitations which will alter the demands made upon said equipment? What new kinds of equipment or new functions will need to be performed, or what kind of control technique needs to be applied?

The same thing goes for the Mars mission. If you can get there in two weeks, the question is: Can you stay two weeks longer or can you stay two years longer, or can you have a permament colony that will stay there indefinitely?

The question is not to determine what are the requirements for a two-year period or for any specific length of time, but to determine from the human point of view: How much farther can any given assignment be stretched? What are the limitations, or what are the requirements other than the need for engineering solutions to those requirements?

REYNOLDS: I would have given a slightly different answer. If I were being asked as a NASA representative, which I do not think I am at this Conference—that just happens to be where I am employed; I am here for a different reason—but if I were here for that reason, and therefore speaking about the fact that NASA is providing funds to support this Conference, it would not be because we want this Conference to specifically answer some design problems that we now are faced with.

We have had the feeling in this and some other fields that an area of scientific interest, usually a rather broad one covering a variety of fields, was one that in the course of time we were going to have to draw on, and we would like to see what can be done to help promote activity in that field.

One of the things to do is to support conferences on interdisciplinary subjects, and another is to support research in such interdisciplinary subjects, not to give particular answers, but just to provide a background that will be available for future use.

SCHWEIGERT: I would like to take a crack at trying to clarify what Dr. Schwarz was getting at. You men are trying very hard to relieve our apprehensions. I am staying about on a plateau on apprehension.

To give a very simple example, some of us might be asked about the concern for rancidity developing in food products and its relation to nutritional quality during a flight. We need to know something about the oxygen situation. We need to know temperatures. We need to know humidities and times—

K. SCHWARZ: Radiation.

SCHWEIGERT: . . . radiation—a whole series of interrelated things, in order to comment intelligently on the question.

Well, maybe you do not want us to comment on the question, but that has something to do with the diet and the kind of food you are going to .put on this flight, and I for one do not know those baselines.

RAHN: On the other hand, there may be some of us who are not nutrition people who would like to have you point out to us the problems, as you did just now, so we can find out how radiation affects rancidity.

Dr. Fremont-Smith, I am wondering whether the word "brainstorming" is the word you want in this Conference.

FREMONT-SMITH: Well, perhaps, except that this has a technical meaning. It is a little bit different. In brainstorming, as I understand it, nobody criticizes anybody else's remark. People just pour out what comes into their minds. Here we do want to have some genuine critique.

REYNOLDS: It just seems to me that this discussion we are having, especially the last comment, indicates the value of an interdisciplinary discussion in this area. It may be that some particular answers to some of these questions will emerge.

RAHN: I will tell you all about the oxygen tensions, and you will tell me all about the rancidity factors.

CALLOWAY: As a point of departure on which we can all perhaps agree, the special problems of human life in outer space stem from the absence of breathable atmosphere and gravitational force and the potential hazards of temperature and radiation exposure. The problems that have arisen in the short-term flights have reflected the consequences of inadequate solutions to them and, perhaps, of the psychosocial climate. Those of us who are more committed to the man than to the mission or the machine note with regret that little has been gleaned from the early flights that will help us to estimate probable long-term metabolic and psychic events.

Experience from the Mercury and Gemini Flights

From the Mercury series we learned that astronauts lose weight during a mission, and that they do not willingly eat and drink enough, and that there may be some cardiovascular decompensation to which the dehydration must surely contribute. The Gemini series has so far confirmed these observations and added the fact that there is x-ray evidence of decreased density of cancellous bone, suggesting loss of skeletal mass, a postulated effect of weightlessness. There has not been so much as a complete 24-hour urine collection and controlled food intake has not been a requirement of any mission. The crews have not been fed the space diet continuously before or after a flight to establish control metabolic values against which subsequent performance could be evaluated. To be fair, the record must show that there are individuals with NASA—both at headquarters and at the Manned Spacecraft Center—who share our concern about the necessity for evaluating human performance, apart from establishing limits of tolerance to a make-shift environment.

So much for history. Let us get on with—

REYNOLDS: I am going to try to fill a peculiar role, that of defending the very things that I fight all the time in my job. I would like to represent either a devil's or angel's advocate here for NASA, and try to give you somewhat of the picture, looking at it from the other side.

The Mercury and the early Gemini missions have required very rapid development of an entirely new kind of technological capability. There have been a tremendous number of things that people have suggested ought to be done while this is going on—a tremendous range of things. Of course, everybody's proposal is the thing that he sees as the most important, because it is the most important to him.

However, the primary and overriding consideration has had to be the overall success, the completion of the mission as such: getting the man up, keeping him there for a prescribed length of time, and getting him safely back down and back home.

The one big edge that we have had internationally is that the whole thing has been done in a goldfish bowl. It is obvious that there are no secrets. The mistakes show up just as everything else, and this has been a part of the planned policy on this program. It has not been, by the way, the easiest thing in the world to contend with. It would have been a lot easier to have done things much more secretly.

The net result of all this is that the things that contribute directly to overall mission success in the way I just defined it have been subjected to a very high degree of what is called quality and reliability assurance, which increases the cost of any individual operation somewhere between two and four times. The things which have not contributed directly to mission success, but have been "add ons," so to speak, have not been subjected to this kind of a testing and a lot of them have failed as a result. An example of this is the fact that we have so few urine specimens from these flights. There is no question but that if somebody had really gone into this carefully and had worked out the system, the urine could have been brought back, but it did not have the direct bearing on the mission success, so it assumed a second priority.

I think an important element here is the fact that the purposes of this manned flight program are in the process of change right now. One is in the approaches to the experiments that are being taken in the headquarters office in Manned Space Flight, where additional people and money are now being allocated to these problems. The selection process has gone on for scientist astronauts; unfortunately there are not many life scientists in this group, but this is not the fault of the selection procedure. Requirements for quality and reliability assurance on experiment hardware have been introduced, so that you can expect as high a reliability of success in the experiments as of the total system in the future.

So there are a number of things that bode well for the future. I am not by any means saying that continuing pressure from individuals such as those represented here to see that good science is done is no longer needed, because I think it is needed; but I think the picture is not quite as black as it may look at first glance.

FENN: Thank you very much.

CALLOWAY: The first metabolic experiment scheduled is GT-7, so we will see the evidence.

REYNOLDS: There is one point you made, Dr. Calloway, that I would like to amplify. You said that enough water was not taken by the astronauts, and I think it ought to be made clear that there was water available. As a matter of fact, they were scheduled to drink a certain amount, and they refused to do so.

CALLOWAY: Water has always been sent along on the missions. When the fuel cells are generating water as a byproduct, then it could be used profitably to reconstitute dried foods. Since most ot the weight of foods is water, use of dehydrated foods permits a major saving of weight. In recent Gemini flights, a freshwater supply was carried and water from the fuel cells was stored. Whether it can be used at present, I do not know, and I think it is a question a bacteriologist would like to take up, or a toxicologist.

POLLARD: Would you describe how a fuel cell works?

ARNOLDI: I can describe it in fairly crude terms. I will try to do it by analogy.

A fuel cell is essentially the equivalent of a storage battery. If you use a battery as a supplier of power—I am not talking about a lead cell battery, but the general category of storage batteries—you may supply power from the chemical energy stored in the storage battery, under circumstances where the decomposition of certain compounds and formation of others, usually consuming electrode materials, will permit you to extract electrical energy. Solid materials may be consumed, and gases evolved, or vice versa.

If you reverse the process and put in energy, this involves reversing the chemical processes which take place in the battery. Electrolysis of water, for example, uses electrical energy to decompose water into hydrogen and oxygen. In Gemini the battery action is the reverse of water electrolysis, combining hydrogen and oxygen and forming water, and obtaining the free energy of that reaction in the form of electrical power.

I have just stated a generality. You can go into more detail and describe the problems of accomplishing this at an electrode, in order to bring gas into a cell and have it react properly at the electrode, a triple interface involving the gas, the electrode surface, and the electrolyte—it is a rather complex engineering problem. It involves the problem of providing just the right kind of an active chemical surface on which to have this reaction take place.

The same thing happens at both electrodes. At one electrode hydrogen is involved, and at the other electrode oxygen is involved. The two processes are matched together by the electrical balance required in the cell.

I am not sure that I am addressing myself properly to your question—

POLLARD: I know more about it than I did before.

REYNOLDS: Hydrogen and oxygen are carried along in cryogenic storage, and the amount that is released from each of the tanks is supposed to be regulated in order to control the flow to the cell.

The water that is generated is theoretically good for drinking, but it has appeared to have several contaminants in it, so that it is not quite certain yet that it is going to be fully potable. However, I think in the biosatellite flights that the water from the fuel cells is going to be used to support the animals.

CALLOWAY: We have been trying to get samples of fuel-cell water to use in reconstituting dehydrated foods. While it may not be delightful it is probably not worse in flavor than that of Army purification tablets in ditch water used to reconstitute combat foods.

Later, when you get into the recovery of urinary water and respiratory water, there will be problems of aesthetics to cope with.

KRAUSS: Are fuel cells now agreed upon as the standard source of energy for future flights?

REYNOLDS: Not for all the flights. The usefulness of a fuel cell is limited in terms of how much cryogenic storage you can afford. They probably are not good for planetary flights, at least according to the present length of time it takes to get to planets; but for a month or two they are all right.

MAYER: Was there not some thought that for longer flights either solar energy or a small reactor would be used, and that fuel cells would have only an intermediate type of use?

KRAUSS: What is the contaminant in the water?

REYNOLDS: The fuel cell is internally a honeycomb of metal surfaces bonded, I think, with phenolic resins, and you tend to get very small quantities of these various materials picked up in the water.

K. SCHWARZ: Could those not be removed very easily by passing them through a very small amount of ion-exchange resin?

REYNOLDS: Well, this is the kind of thing that is being done now.

MAYER: Was there not some thought of having some sort of monitoring device to see if there was any trace of metal contamination? If it was going to be used, obviously you would have to have a whole system of gadgetry to make sure that the water is pure.

REYNOLDS: That is right

EPSTEIN: Why did the astronauts refuse to drink?

REYNOLDS: They said they were not thirsty.

MAYER: Is the problem not that there was no understanding on their part that thirst was a relatively sluggish phenomenon, and that actually, working in very hot conditions, you can become quite dehydrated before you get thirsty. If you have a situation where you are very hot, and it is dry, dehydration is much more rapid—too rapid for thirst to occur.

BROWN: I think there is probably another reason too. There is a bit of folklore to the effect that if you do not drink a lot of water, you will not have the elimination problem, and supposedly this was rather inconvenient.

CALLOWAY: They also do not like the arrangements for defecation which is one of the reasons that there is so much emphasis on a low-residue diet. The men have been fed a conventional low-residue diet for some days before they take off on the flight. I understand that the process is so unattractive that some of the men have asked to have administered an agent to suppress peristalsis.

FREMONT-SMITH: It sounds to me as if Mr. Webb was quite right, that these were human beings exhibiting human factors—psychological and emotional factors—just as one would expect they would. They just did not turn out to be little machines, and therefore could not be expected to react like little machines.

I think this is really worth emphasizing. This enters in at every phase of the program, and I think it is being systematically ignored; not by Mr. Webb, I am glad to say.

TAPPEL: I would like to ask the question if these men were educated in physiological and nutritional problems. It seems to me that they were not educated in the biological necessities of life.

CALLOWAY: I do not know but it is perhaps the case that no amount of instruction before they go up is particularly effective on matters that they think are highly personal or pretty much the business of little old ladies anyway—you know: Did you brush your teeth, and did you eat your vegetables. . .

FREMONT-SMITH: This is the human factor.

MAYER: Some of the instruction that ought to be done in terms of hunger, thirst, and so on, is impossible, because they literally do not have time.

CALLOWAY: I do not believe that, really.

They are thoroughly schooled in such things as survival. They have plenty of time to go out and claw their way through the jungle. I think it is a question of shared perception of priority on the part of the astronauts and the responsible staff.

Food Supplies

EPSTEIN: Could I ask, if we could go back for a minute, about the food: Was the diet acceptable to the astronauts? Did they comment on it?

CALLOWAY: Oh, indeed they did! I believe that the astronauts are permitted to select among the items that are mission-qualified, so that they have some opportunity to eliminate particularly disliked items from the roster.

BROBECK: Do they eat these foods before they go up, or is this the first time they are exposed to them?

CALLOWAY: No, they have eaten them before.

BROBECK: For how long? About two weeks, or something like that?

CALLOWAY: I think not that long.

EPSTEIN: Do they eat all the food?

CALLOWAY: No. McDivitt and White were only about one meal behind in GT-IV, and they said that they were hungry and enjoyed eating and felt better after they ate, but this is not the usual behavior.

There has been very little printed—maybe it is not printable—from the astronauts themselves about these food materials, but then they have not eaten them very long either.

POLLARD: Are these foods sterilized before they are dehydrated?

CALLOWAY: No. The freeze-dried items are cooked, so the amount of handling after cooking sets the level of contamination.

Food Variety Versus Formula Diets

MAYER: There is a curious idea, I think, that diversity of foods is terribly important, particularly in a short period. I have not had any experience with feeding astronauts, but I have had experience with feeding men in combat for months and months and months, and the normal reaction of people who are under stress is to select those items which they like and throw away everything else, and basically, let us say, for the three or four weeks of the Battle of Cassino, where people were feeding exclusively on K rations, or just about, the use of K rations was probably five or six times what it was supposed to be, simply because people took the one or two items they liked, and threw away everything else.

I would imagine that in a situation like space it would be very much more important to find out exactly what it is that each individual likes, and let him have it, rather than really keep on trying to find (through the pressure, I think, to a certain extent, of so many different people and organizations concerned that want to have a part in it) as many items as are palatable, as will be accepted. Somehow this does not ring true for people under stress.

CALLOWAY: How would you react to a formula, then? I do not care what sort of formula you postulate, but let us say something that has no familiar connotations.

EPSTEIN: You mean a liquid diet? Is that what you mean by formula?

CALLOWAY: Just something that on cue you eat or drink a glass of, instead of normal foods.

BROBECK: How about a milkshake, which is not only familiar, but a highly preferred food among most men?

BARNES: Extensive experience with formula diets has now been obtained and, in general, they are satisfactory and well received. The use of everyday foods in space travel may have a public relations value, but from a practical standpoint, specifically processed conventional foods are not necessary. Nutritional quality and acceptability can be achieved in formula-type diets.

CALLOWAY: Men live on formulas for very long periods of time. Our subjects complain all the time, but captive groups such as students, patients, always do complain about food.

The argument for *food* that has been raised—for food as compared to formula—is that this is the only morale item that can be given. I wonder if the present diet *is* a morale item under these conditions.

MAYER: I think that people forget that not only is the variety of food not particularly important, as long as people are under stress—on very long, monotonous flights it might be an entirely different matter—but the maintenance of caloric balance is not by itself that important either, even for periods of one, two, or three weeks.

For instance, it is well known that men in combat are not by and large in caloric balance, and one of the main reasons you need to pull them out of the front lines is not just to get them to rest from constant bombardment, but also in order for them to make up the caloric deficit that they have incurred, in the presence of unlimited amounts of food that they did not feel like consuming. If you get them out of the front lines, those boys will consume 5000 or 6000 calories per day, and then they can go back in.

The idea that people have to be carried in caloric balance at all times does not correspond with anything in human experience. They must have oxygen and water, but food—the caloric balance—can oscillate quite a bit without any damage.

FREMONT-SMITH: The whole evolutionary process has not kept people in this kind of balance.

POLLARD: Consistent with the psychological factor, is it inconceivable to have a staggered diet to which you can add various flavors?

CALLOWAY: This is the formula approach, is it not? You have a formula that provides for nutritional needs and flavor it at will. What you are suggesting is that the astronauts should take along a whole battery of essences and add them as they see fit?

POLLARD: That is right.

WARD: I have seen and had the opportunity to sample most of the so-called space diets and have often wondered about their necessity. The bite-sized cubes generally taste like compressed sawdust or worse and the liquid diets are little better than Pablum. Why cannot they have more or less normal food? The dehydrated foods are generally very acceptable; however, the bouillon-like cubes being used in the Manned Orbiting Laboratory simulator flights are something else again. Are the cubes to be reconstituted or eaten as such?

CALLOWAY: Eaten as such.

WARD: Balanced nutrition is one thing, but I do not really understand the point, not being a nutritionist, of why we are putting these things in such weird forms.

CALLOWAY: Part of the problem is the need to fit 2800 calories in about 100 cubic inches of storage space, per man-day.

FREMONT-SMITH: And this was not determined by nutritionists or by psychologists?

CALLOWAY: No.

FREMONT-SMITH: I think this illustrates the point that we have got to have an interdigitation between the biologists, the psychologists, and the engineers in their original planning, and not have the human factors squeezed into a slot which is predetermined in size, shape, temperature, and so forth, without any serious consideration of the psychological and human needs of the astronaut.

MAYER: Is it not true that the real problem is that you do not want any crumbs in the cabin?

CALLOWAY: That is one of the problems. Another has been power for refrigeration and for heating, as well as weight and stability.

MAYER: Actually, when you have very little space, as you do right now, until we get bigger boosters, the engineers do the best they can. It seems to me that a liquid diet enables you to take advantage of all sorts of odd shapes, nooks, and crannies, because you do not have problems of fitting things.

ARNOLDI: May I suggest one other factor that limits the kind of foods and packaging used—and that is not only the necessity for avoiding crumbs, but also of avoiding contaminant vapors or gases. That limits the contents of the food packages. It means that you cannot have frying fats, you cannot cook a meal, certainly, and you cannot use many condiments that might be acceptable in a restaurant but would represent toxic contaminants in a confined space.

BROBECK: I would like to ask why they cannot tidy up the place with a vacuum hose when they get finished? Are they near the limit of the gas supply and pressure systems in these capsules, so they could not afford to waste a few cubic inches of air?

LIVINGSTON: They have got a high vacuum outside, if they want to use it.

ARNOLDI: You would get too much air with it—too much atmosphere. You could recirculate the atmosphere. You could have a vacuum cleaner with a porous bag, for example. The power that it takes would be pretty small, but the bulk of the piece of equipment would be hard to stow into an already volume-limited capsule. It means one more experiment left behind, for example.

BROWN: Such gadgets have been designed. They have not been used for the reason given—space.

K. SCHWARZ: I would like to make one comment which I should have made earlier.

The idea of comparing combat conditions to conditions in the space capsule strikes me as probably not quite accurate. It is true that you do not need to watch out for caloric balances in combat, but I think you have to watch out very carefully caloric balances in a space capsule, at least if this is going to go on for more than a week, I would say.

So where are we? Do we discuss very short missions, or do we discuss missions which go on for more than a week or a month?

RAHN: I would like to comment as a complete outsider in this area, but I was very much impressed with the comments that Dr. Mayer made a while ago. It seems to me that you are making these poor astronauts subject to fancy experiments. For short missions you can give more ordinary foods, and whether he likes it or not, he will accomplish his mission.

Nobody ever worried about the trapper up North. He had pemmican and tea and that is what he ate until he came to the end of his long trap line.

It seems to me that with the equivalent of pemmican and tea our astronaut would perform a week's mission. Naturally, he would complain about his food, but he would get his job done. It is only when you get to long missions that food selection becomes increasingly important. Now please criticize.

CALLOWAY: If you do not now know about the short mission, you are never going to know about the long one.

RAHN: For the last three years all I have heard about was the seven pounds of water that Cooper lost. Everybody was upset; well, I have never been upset about it. I have worked in the desert, and you can lose seven pounds of water, and there is nothing to it, because this is voluntary dehydration. This is what a man under stress in the desert will do. Cooper was under stress in the heat, and naturally he did not want to drink. Twenty-four hours later he will make it up.

EPSTEIN: Is there not a deterioration in performance? This is not a trapper here, who can take half a day off. This is a man in space.

RAHN: A man in space is just like a soldier in the desert. He will deteriorate in performance, but he will accomplish his job if he has the proper initiative and emotional attitude toward the problem.

MUNRO: Every long flight is preceded by a short flight. In other words, the initial takeoff and stress of that must be part of the longer one, so that all these effects—these immediate effects—will be part of the longer program as well.

If he is going to rehydrate himself later on, he is going to do it in space this time, and not on the ground. All these compensations have to take place subsequently during the travel into outer space.

K. SCHWARZ: I would like to say something to your point.

Strickly from an experimental point of view we know quite a number of essential dietary factors, the deficiency of which can be shown within two or three days. Their absence will cause very acute and fatal damage.

For instance, choline is necessary in the rat. You will see a deficiency after four or five days, if you watch carefully, and it can kill an animal within eight or nine days.

I think you want to watch very carefully and make sure that an organism gets, even for one week, what it needs daily—at least of those dietary elements which we know can be shown to be necessary on short notice. Choline is just an example. The man in space may be very much better off to get those things.

RAHN: I appreciate those things, but we are talking about all these fancy foods that have to be mixed. It seems to me that if I had given that man a big sausage—which does not crumble in space, I guess—and a bag of tea, he would have performed that mission.

CALLOWAY: Yes, but what would happen on the next longer mission?

MAYER: I would question, actually, whether you can test acceptability of long-term menus through short terms, because the problem is entirely different.

Again, I do not have any experience in space, but I did spend 18 months in Libya, which was pretty monotonous in terms of environment, and I was struck by the fact that we had the same food morning, noon, and night—essentially corned beef—and this was acceptable even though I think none of us would choose corned beef for a single meal.

This is what we would choose, probably, any of us who have had experience for very long periods. In other words, a food which is acceptable week after week after week is a very different type of food from the sort that you will choose if you are going to have rotation within a week. You could have rice, probably. I am not terribly fond of rice, but if I know I am going to be on one food for six months, I might choose to have rice as essentially the main constituent of that food.

Unless one is prepared to continue a mad rotation of food for eight months, I think the testing of how long people can be satisfied on a relatively monotonous diet, and what sort of monotonous diet will be satisfying is an entirely different problem from testing the acceptability of 25 different components, each one on a short-term basis. I like oysters; I like *paté de foie gras,* but I would not choose them as a steady diet. And yet I would prefer them to other foods for the next week.

BROBECK: This is the point about the pemmican, because it has been tested the hard way and shown to be acceptable for a long period of time. We are to mix up something in a laboratory in this program, hand it to a man, and say: This is your pemmican.

CALLOWAY: It is known that arctic explorers will eat pemmican. It is known—by tests, anyway—that troops will not always do so.

People who like pemmican eat it a lot, and the same is true of corned beef, probably. But military studies indicate that even given a limited amount of food—a thousand calories a day in a field survival situation—if there are nonpreferred items, the men will not even take in the 1000 calories.

So if you do not want to generalize to years from weeks, I do not want to generalize from one man to men, either.

SCHWEIGERT: I think one of the key factors being brought out here is the significance, or the relative significance, of the quality attributes of the foods. We are using the term "nutrition," but we are looking for quality attributes of foods such as flavor, color, texture, as well as nutritive value and wholesomeness, which means the microbiological and chemical safety. It is apparent that factors of texture and flavor and color very often outweigh nutritive value in the acceptability of food on the short-term consideration. These are all the complexities of factors of which we have words to describe, but very often very poor scientific, objective measurements to elaborate on them, and that is one of the communication problems in this field, I think.

TAPPEL: I think another thing to say about the food problem is that, as Dr. Schweigert has pointed out, we desire the main attributes of the food. The military have long realized this, and they have evolved a food system over a long period of years, as Dr. Calloway can point out, which aims to supply a very similar type of diet to what persons are used to, and hence you get these freeze-dried items for the Gemini flight that are very similar to the Quartermaster Corps' end products for combat feeding. I think it is interesting to note that this probably has gone through 30 years of food research, and this is the best product that has been produced.

I think there is a real need to step up food research in this direction. There is very little being done, as compared to the hardware research.

II. THE MACRONUTRIENTS

Discussion Leader:

DORIS HOWES CALLOWAY
Department of Nutritional Sciences
University of California
Berkeley, California

CALLOWAY: Traditionally, nutritionists are accustomed to thinking in terms of protein, minerals and vitamins; and of their provision in adequate amounts in diets made up of a wide variety of acceptable foods. Even the elemental composition of most of these foods is unknown, let alone the specific compounds into which the elements are organized. Once identified, few of these compounds prove to be "known" physiologically. We do know that traditional diets are not always nutritionally ideal and their improvement is rewarded by gains stature and vigor—until their overconsumption again results in decreased fitness.

Nutritional support of life in space, as it is now visualized, may require dependence on one or two unconventional or even yet-to-be-synthesized food-like materials as the major source of energy, and even the most optimistic outlook envisions transportation and long-term storage of a limited array of highly processed foods. This situation should be ideal for finding out in a practical fashion what things must be included in the diet and what things cannot be, at least in unlimited amount over the long-term. It is in exactly this way that some of our accepted nutritional truths came to be known: the presence of goitrogenic substances and anticoagulants in plants, the need for several of the trace minerals and their toxicity and imbalance relationships, to give only a few examples. Much research will be necessary if we are to avoid this kind of learning experience after the men have passed the point of no return on a Mars mission.

We must decide what criteria of adequacy will be used to judge where the floor and ceiling are to placed with respect to the various substances present in the diet. How do we know when deficiency or excess changes from a just-not-noticeable difference to a just-noticeable one? The Arctic explorer who made it to the Pole on pemmican and tea had only to withstand the rigors of cold and hard work and limited companionship, and that only for a brief period. The astral pioneer must process data and operate complex equipment, endure near-maximal changes of acceleration and G-force, risk radiation exposure, and exercise the highest cognitive skill in carrying out our experiments as well as his own—and he must do it for years.

If we are to travel with a do-it-yourself kit, we must be able to close the material balance. This means that we must know how much is lost from the body, in what forms and by what routes. It also means trapping a number of things we normally ignore in classical nutrition studies, and their systematic analysis. Such chores are often tedious, and unrewarding until the parts fall into fit in a larger context at a later time. Is anything or everything for which we cannot now account sequestered within the body?

Doctor Schwarz will take up the question of micronutrients in a later session; now we are enjoined to discuss the macronutrients. I have chosen to limit this discussion to the energy-yielding constituents of the diet, composed mainly of carbon, hydrogen, oxygen, nitrogen and sulfur. We might wish it were different, as observed by Warren Miller in *Looking for the General:* [2]

"There is something gross about the carbon atom. It will combine with anything. How interesting to consider what we might have been had we been made of silicons instead: a generally cleaner animal, I should think, less given to flatulence, enlarged pores, rumbling innards, calluses, scaly skin, dry scalp, and the stuff that forms in creases and between toes." But for the present we are stuck with carbohydrate, fat and protein.

Before we begin our deliberations, however, I wonder if David Schwarz might tell us something of the results of a human experiment in which nearly pure substances were fed for an extended period. This could serve usefully as a starting point for both this discussion and the one on micronutrients and to my knowledge there have been only two brief reports published so far.[3,4]

Chemically Defined Diet

D. SCHWARZ: My connection with defined diets goes back to the mid-1950's when our company was supplying some of the intermediates for the chemically defined diets being developed by Dr. Jesse Greenstein at the National Cancer Institute. It seemed to me then, and I have had no reason to change this view, that defined diets offered opportunities for controlled studies on intact animals and man with much less ambiguity and much greater possibility for revealing subtle interactions than had been possible previously. The application of defined diets to problems of nutrition in manned space flight and as a model system in working toward a recycling minimum ecological loop for long missions seems to me a fairly obvious outgrowth of the interest aroused in these earlier associations. For the past three years our company has been conducting research on the formulation, stability and biological efficiency of defined liquid diets for NASA, using the rat as our principal test animal. We also supplied the purified amino acid and other key ingredients for liquid diets used in a human feeding trial sponsored by NASA and are currently evaluating the analyses of urine and feces collected during certain phases of these human feeding trials. As I understand it, it is about the latter which you wish me to comment particularly.

From September 1963 to early March 1964 a human feeding trial using chemically defined diets as the sole source of nutrition was conducted under NASA sponsorship at the California Medical Facility in Vacaville, California. There were originally 24 prisoners selected for this study and 15 of them remained with the experiment over its entire term of about six months.

During the last two months of these trials a number of experimental variations were made, including seven days of nitrogen depletion followed by two weeks of repletion, which was in turn followed by step-wise replacement of the pure L-amino acids in the diet by whole protein (beef peptone) and then by a final stage in which the formula diet was replaced by a more or less normal soft diet. In this last two-month period, all urine and feces was collected, measured, and aliquot samples were preserved by freezing. We are now in the process of evaluating the results of analyses of these samples to determine whether there were any gross abnormalities in excretion patterns. So far, we have completed preliminary analysis on the urines only. I have a copy of our preliminary report to NASA here with me in case any of you would like to see the numbers in greater detail. All of the urine analyses were carried out under the supervision of Dr. Samuel Natelson, then at Roosevelt Hospital in New York.

I should like to make it clear that although NASA turned over to us all of the records which were available to them, our role has been one of evaluators after the fact, which makes it particularly desirable that this preliminary report be both conservative and general in its conclusions.

Although we did not have urine and feces specimens from the first four months of the feeding trials, the daily histories, records of weight and other physical measurements, and certain other data were made available to us. Also, a report was published by Dr. Winitz and co-workers,[3] summarizing analyses of blood samples taken from these subjects during the first four months. You will find comment to that paper in *Nutrition Reviews* for August 1965.[5] The gist of Winitz' report is that levels of blood constituents remained within normal range. There was a drop in serum cholesterol when glucose was the principal source of carbohydrate in the diet, which rose when the glucose was replaced by sucrose during a three week period.

Our evaluation of the urine analyses did not disclose any significant abnormalities in the excretion patterns. However, the amount of free amino acid found in the urine would indicate that further improvements can be made either in the amount or balance of the amino acids provided in the diet.

After an initial drop during the first weeks of the trials, all of the subjects seemed to maintain weight well. Taken in its entirety, the feeding trial demonstrates that chemically defined diets can supply adequate nutrition for humans for a period of six months—and the indications are that this could have been continued considerably longer. An important finding is the fact that fecal dry solids averaged only three to four grams per day per man. Eliminations occurred rather irregularly at from two- to five-day intervals. Returning to the soft diet did not appear to present any serious problems, though it did immediately result in a significant increase in fecal output.

We think that this experiment demonstrates that chemically defined diets (or formula diets patterned after them) are practical and safe for extended use as the sole source of nutrition for humans. Much valuable experience was gained through these trials. Human nutrition experiments of this type generate enormous numbers of samples. (Approximately 50,000 individual assays have been performed on the urine samples collected in the final two months.) Even with the benefit of this experience, it is clear that future experiments of this type will require the most careful prior planning and control. In spite of the formidable logistics, I believe that detailed studies using defined diets and formula diets will be essential for gaining the understanding of minimum nutritional requirements which NASA ultimately need for life support on extended missions.

Carbohydrates and Serum Cholesterol

MOSSEL: We have all been impressed in contintental Europe by the studies of Winitz, saying that these experimental human guinea pigs getting synthetic diets had very low serum cholesterol levels of 150 mg. percent, and when you reached glucose by sucrose it went up to 235. Is it not worthwhile in this era of coronary disease, to take this up and spend five minutes on this subject?

Would anyone feel that that nutrition finding has any interpretation? What is it that causes this rise in serum cholesterol so significantly when you replace glucose by sucrose in this synthetic diet?

MAYER: There have been several papers. For example MacDonald finds that the replacement of starch by sucrose in very large amounts considerably increases all blood lipids, including blood cholesterol in men, but that it has very little effect in women, showing once again that there is a difference between men and women.[6]

FREMONT-SMITH: *Vive la différence!*

MOSSEL: There is also a significant difference in the morbidity and mortality in cardiovascular diseases between men and women, so I think this is a highly significant study.

MAYER: In general it seems to me that we should not forget that we are dealing with a group of men of an age group where the first cause of death (after accidents), under the best circumstances, is normally coronary catastrophe.

Now, I am obviously, as a nutritionist, very interested in making sure that they do not develop mineral deficiency, but at the same time we must remember that from a nutritional standpoint, from what we know at present, the overwhelming risk is that they might die of something which they might die of outside of their capsule; in particular, coronary catastrophe. This may well be the nutritional problem which really might create the greatest disturbance in space travel.

The one thing that can be said in terms of practical considerations is that, while the differences were very large, they did involve the feeding of what, except perhaps in a sugarcane growing area, would be very unrealistic amounts of sucrose. I have forgotten the exact amounts, but those were very large amounts—perhaps 400 gm. of sucrose a day, versus 400 gm. of starch.

CALLOWAY: Since we are primarily interested in protein questions, in our experiments we deliberately include a variety of carbohydrates and fats, with about 100 gm. of sucrose a day constantly in the diet. The men's serum total cholesterol values fall very promptly, so some sucrose is compatible with normal blood lipid patterns. We cannot account for reduced cholesterol levels in our subjects, except that it has something to do with the experimental situation.

Protein Requirements

We are agreed on the essential role of some of the constituent amino acids of protein and of the polyunsaturated fatty acids that make up the fats, and may dispute the essentiality of carbohydrate as such, or in specific forms. But for purposes of energy we may think in terms of some fat, some carbohydrate and some protein. The question of minimum protein is one that Dr. Munro has dealt with so extensively that I asked him if he would make some comments about what is essential, and if it is desirable to use protein to arrive at carbohydrate.

MUNRO: This question of protein requirements is still quite unsettled in many of its aspects. This, of course, could be said with the word "protein" exchanged for any nutrient which you care about, but it was acutely brought to notice when an attempt was made by the WHO-FAO Committee to revise their booklet on protein requirements of 1957.[7]

In 1965 another group met in Geneva and prepared a report on protein requirements.[8] I was a member of that group. The final point of view taken on how to assess requirements is probably important with regard to stresses and other aspects of space travel which would influence these requirements. We took the attitude that we would try and make a factorial approach (Table 1); that is to say, as in the case of calories we would have the basal requirement, and we would add to that requirements for various purposes.

Now, the first question, then, was selecting a basal need, and we took the ancient observation—which, of course, is very familiar to nutritionists, but perhaps not to our engineering colleagues—of the minimum nitrogen loss from the body, the minimum amount of protein lost from the body, on a protein-free diet.

If your intake of protein is suddenly subtracted, then the nitrogen output in the urine does not go down to zero, but continues to produce a loss (FIGURE 1).[9]

Now, the question is: At what point in this continuously declining output do we choose our level at which we say the subject is now more or less steady?—because he is not really steady.

There are two phases here. The first of them is a rapid phase, and at a point which can be defined in many experiments, this gives place to a more slowly declining phase, a point of inflexion.

This rapid phase is probably associated with the loss of protein from organs such as liver, gastrointestinal mucosa, the pancreas, and some undisclosed places in the carcass which are rapidly lost and regained—in the case

TABLE 1

THE FACTORIAL APPROACH TO ESTIMATING THE PROTEIN REQUIREMENTS OF MAN
(Adapted from WHO Report, 1965 [8])

Component of requirement	Estimated Requirement	
	As nitrogen	As body protein
	mg/kg body weight/day	
Basal urinary N	46	288
Endogenous fecal N	20	125
Dermal N	20	125
Total	86	538
Add 10 percent for everyday stresses	95	594
Range of ± 20 per cent	—	470–710
Replacement by dietary protein with a net protein utilization value of 80	—	740
Range of ± 20 per cent		590–890

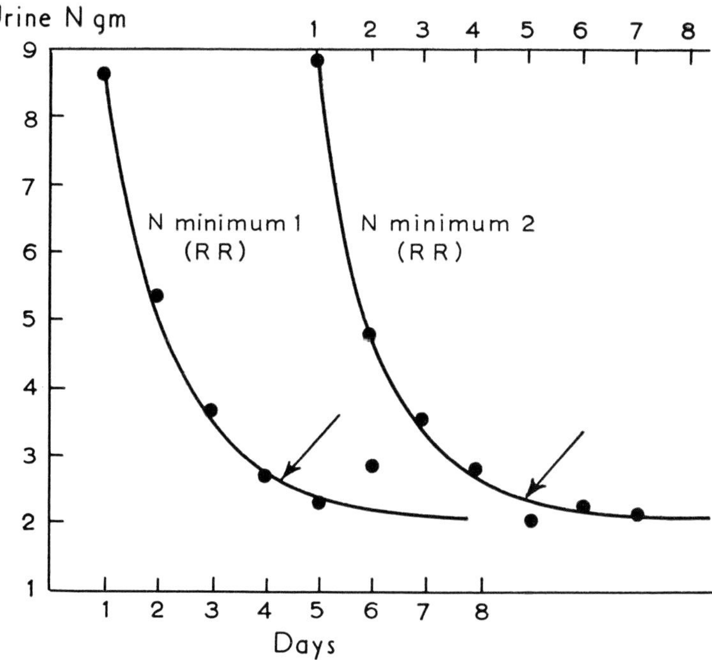

FIGURE 1. Urinary nitrogen excretion of a human subject during two different periods on a proteinfree diet. The point of inflexion, indicating loss of the most labile body nitrogen, is shown by an arrow. (Reproduced from Martin & Robinson, 1922.)[9]

of the liver, within an hour or two there are changes in protein synthesis and protein content which are measurable.

We regarded these changes as so transient and labile that they were not in fact part of our requirement problem. They represent metabolic fluctuations.

At the point of inflexion—shown by arrows in the Figure—which take place in the rat at about three days—perhaps a little longer in man—the loss of nitrogen in the urine represents continuing breakdown of more important tissue constituents. Notably here we begin to lose measurable amounts of muscle protein.

So this point was regarded as the basal output of nitrogen in the urine, and any diet has to be capable of replacing this loss of body protein.

The figure which was assessed for this was 46 milligrams per kilo per day, which is equivalent to an amount of body protein per day—not dietary, but *body* protein of 288 mg./kg. of body weight/day, obtained by multiplying the calculated endogenous urinary N by 6.25.*

* Most protein contains 16% of nitrogen so the reciprocal factor of 6.25 is used to convert nitrogen to average protein. Ed.

In addition to urinary basal nitrogen loss, you have, of course, obligatory fecal nitrogen, which we placed at 20 mg. per day, i.e., 125 mg protein/kg, and a loss of cutaneous nitrogen, which was from the literature assessed at that same level—that is, 125 mg. of protein/kg. The total of these adds up to 590 mg.; that is 0.59 gram of protein per kilogram.

I will comment on some of these points later. In the meantime, let's go on and see what additional requirements we had to achieve before we considered our subjects to be normally nourished.

The stresses of everyday life were brought in as a component; the stresses of anxiety, minor infections, and other causes of increased adrenocortical activity, which were considered to give rise to losses which were then replaced when the subject was no longer under stress, and this was put at 10 percent of the total body protein requirement. That is to say, a replacement requirement of 9 mg. of nitrogen, representing a loss of 55 mg. of protein per kg. body weight. The total requirement, including the 10 percent addition for stress, thus becomes 594 mg. protein per kg. body weight per day (Table 1). These figures are mathematically accurate, but they obviously have a large biological error. The amount of 0.59 of a gram of protein per kilo per day was regarded as the minimum replacement within the body.

Now, in addition we have a subjective range. Individual subjects will not come into equilibrium when this loss is replaced; in some cases they will do so on a lower intake, and in some cases on a higher. From the published evidence the range was taken to be 20 percent.[10] So this means that we have a range from 470 mg. to 710 mg., that is, an average of 0.59 gm. protein per kg. body weight, with a range of 0.47 to 0.71.

When we consider how to replace this body protein loss with dietary protein, we have to recognize that the protein of the average diet is not fully utilized. In the case of Western dietaries containing good quality protein, utilization, as judged by net protein utilization values, is about 80 percent effective. Thus the figure for protein requirement becomes inflated by a factor of 100/80. Our final estimate of how protein should be consumed in the form of a mixed Western-type diet thus becomes 0.74 gm./kg. body weight/day (Table 1). If we assume that individual variation for two standard deviations from this mean value does not exceed 20 percent (0.59 to 0.89 gm./kg.), then we can say that an intake of 0.9 gm. protein/kg./day will be adequate to deal with the protein requirements of 98 percent of the population.

Now, from the point of view of international nutrition, you have to cover the upper limit. If people vary genetically or in other ways which cause them to have a lower or a higher requirement, you have to budget for the upper limit in order to provide a protective figure.

There are a number of points which are relevant to this morning's discussion which we have to consider.

First of all, we have neglected the initial labile material (FIGURE 1) in our calculations. If you vary the protein intake of rats, the amount of protein in the liver is very easily affected. The rat appears to be almost unlimited in its capacity for an increase in protein content of the liver cells. The change occurs rapidly, and similar changes will take place in some other labile organs.

The question is: Does the presence or absence of this additional material in these organs confer any advantages on the animal? Does our estimate, in other words, of 0.9 for the upper limit of protein requirement represent a loss of something less easily defined than we have defined this? Do these organs function more efficiently at higher than minimal protein intakes?

The answer to this is not at all satisfactory. We have no real experimental evidence to demonstrate that these supraoptimal intakes confer benefits subsequently, but I think there may be some discussion on this point.

MAYER: I think—would you not agree Dr. Munro—that it is perhaps not a good idea to get snowed by the apparently precise knowledge that is displayed the minute one puts figures on the board?

The basal nitrogen, that 288 mg. figure, at least the order of magnitude is reasonably well known. Fecal nitrogen data are reasonably good too; cutaneous nitrogen—the data are relatively poor compared to the other two. Those are data obtained on not that many subjects when you come right down to it, and usually of a fairly limited age range. The rest, of course, are estimates, and it is a rather curious thing that one ends up always with the top being very close to a gram per kilogram, which makes it socially acceptable.

The first meeting on requirements was a meeting of the League of Nations, I think in 1931, which was attended by Mellanby and Hazel Stiebeling, my father, André Mayer, and various other people, and they picked the figure of one gram per kilogam as being an acceptable figure, and it has remained so for the upper limit ever since.

If one goes back before that, it seems to me that the discussion as to whether or not the high labile nitrogen is useful goes back to the discussion around 1910 between Voit and Chittenden to the effect that one can maintain people in good health on 120 gm. of protein a day, and therefore this must be a good thing; or, conversely, one can maintain people in good health on 50 gm. per day, and this must be a good thing.

The only data I know of of the usefulness of the labile nitrogen [1] are the data of Allison on toxicity and the use of that labile nitrogen as a protection against intoxication, and the Japanese data on the fact that if one is subjected to any sort of [physical] effort, and life is not smooth, then unless one has this extra labile nitrogen, one tends to make muscle [at the expense] of hemoglobin or do shifts of that sort.

It is very tenuous evidence either way.

MUNRO: Well, this, of course, is the view that we took, that it was so tenuous that we were not justified in adding a quota to take care of it.

BROBECK: I would like to ask a question about this basal nitrogen loss that I have never understood, though I have tried to use this for calculations of the same sort.

It seems to me very likely that the basal loss, which seems to be constant, has the same relation to nitrogen exchange that the basal level for energy exchange does for energy balance. The nutrition people here know this very well, but I will review it very briefly.

If during fasting a man's energy expenditure is 1200 kilocalories a day, and then you say: I'm going to meet this by giving him a diet of such-and-such a composition of 1200 kilocalories, you find that his energy expenditure has gone up to 1400 or 1500. This is what is called a specific dynamic effect, or specific dynamic action.

Are there data about this relative to nitrogen? It seems to me very likely that if a man is turning over 5 gm. of nitrogen during a constant fasting condition, and if you then gave him 5 gm., you might find that he now begins to lose 7 gm. Perhaps the baseline should be the level at which he first comes into a true balance.

CALLOWAY: We just did that.

BROBECK: What did you find?

CALLOWAY: That he does not stay quite in balance when you feed him an amount of high-quality protein equal to his own endogenous output. We measured urinary, fecal and cutaneous nitrogen output at adequate caloric intakes. For most of the young men we studied that value was something like 3.6 grams of nitrogen per day and was not closely correlated with body weight.[12]

We think that a large part of the initial adjustment to changes in protein intake can be accounted for as urea. When protein intake drops, blood urea nitrogen falls, and as the urea space is the same as the total body water, a drop of only 5 mg. percent represents about 2.75 grams of nitrogen. There is also a drop in circulating blood volume which allows removal of serum proteins without any apparent change in concentration.

Loss of sweat nitrogen is related to urea levels in our experiments, which means that body losses vary with dietary intake in this way, also.[13]

BARNES: Dr. Calloway, in your nitrogen balance studies you could get down to levels of intake less than 5.9 gm. nitrogen, could you not, and still maintain nitrogen equilibrium on an NPU-80 protein source?

CALLOWAY: We were using egg albumin as our source.

BARNES: And how far did you go down in nitrogen intake?

CALLOWAY: We went down to 3.8 gm. of total nitrogen, of which 3.28 was protein nitrogen; the rest was casual nitrogen in the diet.

BARNES: And they were in balance at that level?

CALLOWAY: Oh, no.*

BARNES: They were not in balance at that level?

MAYER: That's 22 gm. of protein?

BARNES: Hazel Fox and her associates at the University of Nebraska have measured nitrogen balance in healthy young men.[14] Using cereal proteins, she has found that at about 36 gm. of protein a day a slightly negative balance is obtained and this can be brought back into equilibrium with nonspecific sources of nitrogen.

Now, this is cereal protein, and nitrogen equilibrium is achieved just with the addition of diammonium citrate, or some other nonspecific nitrogen source—pointing out what she believes to be evidence that at low nitrogen intakes, it is nitrogen rather than essential amino acids that are limiting.

MUNRO: This would agree with quite a lot of evidence from other sources. The requirement at low intakes is as much for nitrogen—more for nitrogen than essential amino acids.

BARNES: Well, I mention this here mainly because Dr. Calloway was stressing the point that good, egg protein was used in her studies, whereas the Nebraska group were working with a protein source that would have a much lower value, and still would bring the male subjects into equilibrium at a rather low total nitrogen intake.

MAYER: When you are talking about balance, I think you have to specify, really, what sort of individuals these were. I mean, wheat protein would be a poor protein if you were dealing with growth.

BARNES: This is not growth. We are talking about adults.

CALLOWAY: I think you were about to make the point that the balance of amino acids in wheat protein is respectable for adults.

MAYER: I was just saying cereal protein is not bad, the difference between cereal protein and egg albumin is not that great, if you are dealing with adults.

BARNES: This might be particularly true if you are dealing with an adult human being, and not a rat.

CALLOWAY: I think part of the problem is methodologic, because in experiments of this kind all of the errors summate to predict a more positive balance than actually exists. There are, generally speaking, overestimations of intake and underestimations of output.

So that I think whenever we talk about "near things" in balances—and cutaneous losses are almost never measured except occasionally in Dr. Barnes' laboratory and in our own—that the tendency would be to predict

* Subsequently, we have found one subject who maintained nitrogen balance at that intake, out of 10 studied.

balance at somewhat of a lower intake than actually proves to be the case when you add everything up.

MUNRO: Yes. As you will realize, one errs on the side of safety when predicting for cutaneous and other losses, because it is more serious to be too low than to be somewhat high.

BROBECK: Should we not have the record show that no one here believes that this diet is going to be deficient in protein?

MUNRO: No.

BROBECK: It may have a good bit more protein than is needed, but it is certainly not going to be deficient.

MUNRO: The second point which I wanted to make in regard to this type of factorial approach is that there may be body constituents whose sensitivity to protein levels is important, and is important in the context in which we are discussing them this week.

For example, the sensitivity of bone marrow to protein in the diet has recently been demonstrated. There were published experiments from the Reissman [15] group which paralleled some unpublished data we have ourselves, demonstrating in our case that within this short period—four days in the rat—the capacity of the bone marrow to take up iron is very greatly reduced. If you inject radioactive iron into your animals, after four days of depletion the deposit in the marrow becomes very much smaller due to the absence or diminution of hemopoietic elements—red-cell-forming elements. At the same time the deposition in liver increases, so you have a tissue here which is extremely sensitive.

What we do not know, and what I do not think anybody knows yet, is at what level of protein intake do you achieve a plateau? In other words, if the iron ^{59} uptake is plotted against dietary protein, do you eventually reach a point where the marrow—well, you must reach a point where the marrow is taking up a maximal amount, and then plateaus, and at what point is this related to the level of protein in the diet, and what is our requirement?

This might be important under conditions where low atmospheric pressures cause changes in red-cell production in space flight. The mechanism involved in this case, for those of you who are not biologists, is that the kidney produces the hormone erythropoietin, which stimulates marrow red-cell series production, and that when you inject radioactive iron, the amount which is deposited there or deposited in other tissues, such as the liver, is determined by the amount of erythropoietin in circulation at the time, and this apparently, from the new evidence, is very sensitive to amino acid supply in dietary protein content.

So this could be one factor in assessing the protein requirements in space travel, if in fact the subjects are existing under conditions similar to those of high altitudes and therefore getting the stimulus of erythropoietin secretion which occurs at high altitudes and gives an increased uptake of iron in the marrow, with increased red-cell production.

This merely illustrates one of the many ways in which subtle changes can be taking place in relation to dietary protein level which have still to be explored. The nitrogen balance data are all right as a first approximation, but you never know when another tissue will reveal evidence of sensitivity to protein level.

Dermal and Intestinal Nitrogen Loss

Thirdly, we have to consider the cutaneous nitrogen. Here the problem relevant to space travel is sweating nitrogen loss. The evidence with regard to cutaneous loss was recently added to by Consolazio,[16] and we found it rather difficult to accept his conclusion. What he concluded was that under conditions of heat stress the cutaneous loss of nitrogen through sweat increases, which is acceptable enough, but that this is not carried out by reducing the losses in other directions. You do not transfer to the sweat the nitrogen that you would lose in the urine, and therefore you get a real increase in the nitrogen protein requirements because you have extra loss of nitrogen in the sweat uncompensated by urinary diminution.

Now, this may be an illusion. It may be—and I do not think his experiments exclude the possibility—that the heat stress gives rise to adrenocortical stimulation, and in consequence there is an extra loss of nitrogen generally.

In other words, he is getting a short-term adrenocortical effect due to the heat, a response which is known to occur in animals.

So, therefore, we eventually concluded that the losses due to hot climates and in the present context, in space travel—presumably losses due to heat—would be in effect balanced by reduced urinary nitrogen output.

So much, then, for the cutaneous nitrogen. Then the fourth question which arises is genetic variations in requirements.

EPSTEIN: Can I ask a question here? How are these losses from the skin measured?

MUNRO: Well, sweat is collected over—I think in the Consolazio experiments it was during an eight-hour period, during the day.

EPSTEIN: What portion of the body?

MUNRO: I think he used the arm for this purpose. It is not the total body sweat.

CALLOWAY: Consolazio has predicted from total body water loss using composition from arm sweat values. This can be misleading because arm sweat, collected in a moisture-proof bag, does not have the same composition as sweat collected from some other areas of the body by sweat pads, and by no means matches what we get when we bathe subjects—chemically wash them—before and after a period of sweating induced by exercise. We have not measured sweating under heat stress.

FREMONT-SMITH: Which way do the differences go when you bathe them?

CALLOWAY: Generally less.

FREMONT-SMITH: Less loss than the arm sweat alone?

CALLOWAY: Yes—that is as predicted on the basis of the composition of arm sweat. This is not true for all sweat constituents, however. Our measured losses from the entire body under sedentary, comfortable conditions are somewhat lower than Consolazio's or in the older studies from Dr. Mitchell's laboratory.[17] In the latter case, the men were seated in a hot chamber, on a metal chair with holes in it. There he collected all the sweat, and those losses appeared to be about the same as Frank Consolazio's. But then, again that is heat-induced sweating, which may be different.

EPSTEIN: Does this measurement include the loss from the epidermis?

CALLOWAY: Not in the case of the subjects we washed after short-term exercise without hard scrubbing because they do not accumulate much cellular debris in 10 minutes. We do collect it as part of our longer-term studies, and we do not attempt to separate it out. We also add hair and whiskers and nails to arrive at a total value for integumentary losses.

MUNRO: I should add that the Mitchell experiments [17] were carried out by rubbing down the subject, and there is no doubt that that added something to the desquamation loss, and that this contributed materially, I think, to the very high iron losses which were observed in this study.

MAYER: One of the problems with the factorial method is that the variants might not be independent of intake. For instance, there are data that show that hair length, or hair growth, and fingernail growth may be in turn influenced by protein intake.

CALLOWAY: That is the point I was making with respect to urea. A man on a high-nitrogen diet will lose more nitrogen in his sweat than one on a low-nitrogen diet.

EPSTEIN: If I could just pursue this a moment longer, is the magnitude of loss by desquamation from the epidermis similar to the loss of the intestinal surface?

MUNRO: According to our computations, they were of equal magnitude in terms of endogenous fecal *N*.

EPSTEIN: Is that confirmed by these washing experiments?

CALLOWAY: The value even including scalp hair, whiskers and nails, is by no means anything like what you get from the intestinal tract. Fortunately, you recover most of what you lose from the intestinal tract by the cannibalism of your own sloughed-off cells, whereas everything from the body surface is total loss. The turnover time of the skin cell is nothing like intestinal mucosal turnover rate.

POLLARD: Is there not a big problem in determining fecal loss due to the contributions or deletions by the gastrointestinal microflora?

MAYER: Fecal losses to a certain extent are dependent on the fiber content, the volume of the feces, and so on. The fecal losses are by and large not the proteins that you have consumed, but they are desquamated intestinal cells, bacteria and digestive enzymes.

POLLARD: In other words, what I am gathering from this is that there is not very great accuracy from all of this.

CALLOWAY: That is right. Your question, I suppose, is: If you did not have bacteria there, would you have a smaller fecal loss? Even on protein-free diets, in man the fecal nitrogen is not appreciably lower than it is on a diet containing an adequate supply of protein. The bacteria can use our own mucosal cells and secretions.

MUNRO: Yes, this figure refers to what is known as metabolic fecal nitrogen, the result of the obligatory loss which was just referred to.

K. SCHWARZ: In germ-free animals you have about an equal fecal loss, if I remember correctly—whether you have germs or not.

GUSTAFSSON: This has been studied to some extent, but we do not have the full answer yet.

If one puts a conventional growing rat on a low-protein diet—say, 8 percent casein—ordinarily the rat stops growing. The germ-free rat, however, on the same diet continues to grow. The conclusion would be that the dietary protein in the conventional rat is utilized not only by the host but also by the intestinal flora.

Careful measurements of the input and output of nitrogen in the adult rat, however, have failed to show any major differences between germ-free and conventional rats. On a semisynthetic diet, with a very low fiber content, the utilization of the diet seems to be rather high. There is furthermore no difference in fecal output before and sometime after the germ-free animal has been contaminated with intestinal bacteria from conventional animals. The fecal excretion of nitrogen is higher the first few days after the infection, but after five or six days it reaches the steady state at the same level as before.

To make the situation still more complex, there is about 30 to 50 times higher output of mucins in the germ-free than in the conventional animal.

We have also found recently that some bacteria in the intestinal flora are digested by the host, and some are not. Germ-free animals were kept on a diet, which was very carefully freed of any bacteria to begin with and fed killed bacteria of different strains. The amount of bacteria in the feces was then followed.

In an individual living on a limited protein intake, it could be important what kind of bacterial flora is present in his gut.

MUNRO: May I ask whether coprophagy is excluded in these experiments, and whether it differs in germ-free and conventional animals?

GUSTAFSSON: In the experiments where killed bacteria were fed, coprophagy was prevented, but not in the other experiments which I described.

CALLOWAY: Do germ-free animals practice coprophagy?

GUSTAFSSON: Yes.

FREMONT-SMITH: More than germ-laden animals?

GUSTAFSSON: There is both indirect and direct evidence for this.

There is a delayed turnover of bile acids in germ-free animals. If ^{14}C-labeled bile acid is fed to germ-free animals and to conventional animals at the same time, it is possible to demonstrate that the biological half-life of the bile acid is about two days in the conventional animal and about ten days in the germ-free animal.

This was thought to be due to the absence of the intestinal flora, which in conventional animals metabolizes the bile acids in different ways. When the experiment was repeated with the animals in restrictive units to prevent coprophagy, the half-life of the labeled bile acids was six days in the germ-free animal.

Some of the delayed output of the labeled bile acid is thus due to coprophagy. We have later also demonstrated coprophagy in germ-free animals by feeding rats nondigestible tracers.

Individual Variation

MUNRO: Well, I wanted to go on next to genetic variations, because this is obviously important too. You will recollect, in our report for populations we gave a range and showed the upper limit as being the only safe one to cover 98 percent of the population. This was based on the limited—the very limited number of experiments where an attempt has been made to find out the range of protein requirements of individuals in the population, and the best estimate we could obtain was plus or minus 20 percent. This is largely based on Mitchell's work, published in 1949.[10]

Nevertheless, it does emphasize that there is a range—a probable range—and that it might be desirable at least to consider it and even to make use of it in selecting groups of people for long-term studies in space; namely, that one could perhaps exclude those who were in the upper bracket, if protein was a limiting factor in designing a program.

MAYER: Could I emphasize the point you just made—because it seems to me that one of the things that the people concerned with spacemen ought to know is the fact that all the data we have are data obtained on a relatively limited group of people who tend by and large to be relatively younger men, and that we really do not have any assurance as to how many people are in the upper limit and how far up they may go—whether it is 95 percent or 98 percent that are covered by 1 gm./kg. of protein, or 0.9.

We just do not know, and we really do not know how far up certain individuals may go, so that it is very important for certain experimental situations to obtain the balance data on the individuals that are going to be sent on missions, rather than rely on the idea that we know that 95 percent or 98 percent of people are covered by this or that value for nitrogen, or any nutrients, because, actually, even that much we really cannot tell with a great deal of assurance.

SCHWEIGERT: To put it another way, it would seem that we are very concerned a number of times about reducing the volume for the food 20 percent or 10 percent, or having a higher caloric density food. It would seem to me that you could get at least as much saving right within the protein variable, assuming it would be one of the critical nutrients, as you could by worrying about caloric density per unit volume of food.

MAYER: If you picked the right person, you mean?

SCHWEIGERT: Yes.

POLLARD: You have indicated that about 1 gm. would be necessary for good healthy status. Can man's needs be reduced under such circumstances as hibernation?

MUNRO: This has in fact been suggested during the flight as a means of reducing caloric needs as well as protein. I think it has not reached the stage at which it can yet be exploited seriously.

CALLOWAY: Is it not true, though, that if you put a man into hibernation, that would be maximum physical deconditioning, and therefore you would expect him to have a larger nitrogen loss? The better-trained, more muscular subject will have a larger loss of urinary nitrogen than one who is less fit, when both are limited to sedentary activity.

SCHWEIGERT: This is not necessarily bad, is it?

CALLOWAY: This is a loss of muscle mass, and in the proposed hibernation scheme, it depends on whether you want him to be active as soon as you wake him up—such as putting him in a space suit where he has a fourth of an atmosphere of pressure to operate against, and expecting him to work hard. This involves judgment as to the necessity for all that muscle and all that bone that our culture values.

MUNRO: Another problem is the amount of water required for excreting metabolites in the urine. Therefore, it is of some importance to try to keep the level down if this can be conveniently done.

BROBECK: This impresses me the wrong way, no doubt because of my ignorance; from what I have seen about what these men do, it seems to me that if weight is all this problem, what you ought to do is send up a very bright nine-year-old boy. His weight and everything he needs for support is going to be half or a third what these husky astronauts need. What do they do that he could not do?

CALLOWAY: Dr. Reynolds, how many times have people asked why you did not send midgets?

ARNOLDI: Not very many midgets have qualified as test pilots yet.

JENKINS: The cosmonauts are pretty big guys—90 kilograms.

CALLOWAY: I suppose, Dr. Brobeck, there is not any answer, except that astronauts are selected on the basis of pilot qualifications and other factors than body size.

BROBECK: Yes, but what I am suggesting is that if the thing comes down to being a question of another cubic inch or another gram of nitrogen more or less, you might pick out people simply in terms of size; it would simplify this problem.

BROWN: May I suggest another way of looking at this?

I think we are thinking too much of saving weight in space when we extrapolate into long missions in the future. The payloads we will be flying over the next couple of decades will be just orders of magnitude greater, and the crew sizes orders of magnitude greater also, so if we think of this just as a nutritional problem, then I think something else comes out of these numbers.

The point is that there is a tremendous variation in the population, and it behooves NASA to pay attention to the individual requirements.

Now, there are two ways you can meet this. You can decide that Astronaut X is going to go on a journey, and you can do a long research, find out exactly what his requirements are and meet them. Or you can invest some payload in extra food that you know he is not going to eat, allow him *ad libitum* intake, and assume that he will automatically adjust, given a reasonably familiar diet.

If you are not constrained by payload limitations, is there anything wrong with the latter policy? It seems to me that detailed studies to determine the requirements of an individual astronaut are just prohibitive.

CALLOWAY: If you take that attitude, you are never going to know except in terms of "enough" of everything, which is why we are exactly where we are today. We think we know what people eat. For the Army Master Menu, they buy about 200 different items in one month. We do not know what the composition of these items is. We do not have the foggiest idea of what normal people eat under normal circumstances.

And if we want to go from this to algae or *Hydrogenomonas* or a chemically regenerative system, someday we have to know what these numbers are, whether we use them or do not. We are not saving weight here. We can send calories in the form of protein as well as we could something else.

What we are saying is: Can we set these limits so that we know that if this is what we can provide in a given situation, it is enough, or is there something to be gained by more?

BROWN: Is the individual variation so great that you cannot expect to use average numbers for this purpose? Do you have to do these studies on the astronauts that you are concerned about?

CALLOWAY: Depending on how finely you want to cut the minimum, I would think you would have to.

REYNOLDS: If you do assess thoroughly one individual, preflight, how much confidence can you have that that individual is going to maintain these characteristics under new environmental circumstances?

BROWN: That is the trap that was being set. You would have to do the study in flight.

CALLOWAY: Not only that; let's say you are planning on a three-year flight. To know absolutely whether a given diet is adequate to maintain a group of functions that we have defined as being necessary for this trip, we have to have men on this diet for three years. If you perform the test on astronauts themselves, they are exposed twice as long to the test system you are testing for.

MAYER: I think it is probably a good idea to simply check that they do not have an unusually high requirement for something under short-term conditions.

I mean, you would not have all the answers, but you would be better off than if you assumed that they conformed to the average without any check. That could be done on a relatively short-term basis.

CALLOWAY: There are at least 37 substances that we all agree are required nutrients. So if we tested the astronauts for these one at a time, that is 37 experiments.

BROWN: It may not be useful to worry the point, but it seems to me we have a tremendous amount of experience feeding people, quite a variety of people, flying only about five or six miles above the earth, and we do not know, really, what they eat, but we do know how to keep them reasonably happy with these TV dinners. So we go up to 200 miles, and we are worried about toothpaste tubes filled with peanut butter, and all that kind of thing, and I just cannot believe that the state of the art is not going to advance very rapidly, as the consumer demand builds up on this food.

CALLOWAY: Then you never really need to know what people require, because we can just send anything, willy-nilly, the same as we have been doing here? That is, you feed a mixture of enough corn, soybean oil, meal, and alfalfa to a pig and he grows nicely on it, that is enough; is that what you are saying?

BARNES: It is not just a matter of space that is involved in arriving at some knowledge of minimums in terms of nutrition. It is basic knowledge of nutrition, and it is a basic knowledge of all that is around us in nature, and it has certainly been of considerable importance in agriculture, and it is of importance to the underdeveloped countries of the world, and we can go on and on.

Space happens to be pinpointed at this meeting, but I would hope that we could keep in mind that there is something much broader than space that is involved in this whole topic.

TAPPEL: I would like to second what Professor Barnes said, and that is that we are not responsible just for space flights, but we are responsible for something like four billion people. We do need exact nutritional information, and we do need to know what the averages are for diets under very drastic conditions.

REYNOLDS: Another point, I think, related to this is the fact that I think space and weight are always going to be at a premium in space flight, because it costs so many dollars per pound to launch any kind of an extraterrestrial vehicle. As a result, I think that when it comes to food supply we are always going to be in a position of having to defend concretely the amount of space and weight that is going to be devoted to it.

MAYER: Yes, but I think there are two entirely different problems, depending on whether you are talking about the micronutrients of the diet or the macronutrients, and depending also on whether you are talking about space or whether you are talking about underdeveloped countries.

As far as we know there is no known mechanism that is going to make you overeat of a poor diet in order to get a missing nutrient. By and large, deficiencies tend to work in reverse, by cutting down on the food intake, so that if one is dealing with an underdeveloped country and its population, one is concerned very much with the adequacy of the diet under minimum terms, in terms of making sure that the number of calories that people consume does contain in fact the 37 or 57 nutrients that they require.

Now, when one is dealing with space, the problem is not minimum amounts of vitamins, minimum amounts of trace minerals, and so on, because there it is not going to change anything in terms of the logistics of the operation to add more thiamine or more selenium, or whatever it is. It may, however, make a difference in the logistics of the operation whether you are putting more protein or less protein, more carbohydrate or less carbohydrate, and so on. So all these knowledges are very important, and I hope we get them all, but they are all unequally relevant to the problem of space or to the problem of underdeveloped countries in terms of practical operations.

MUNRO: Could I make it quite clear what I am attempting to do? This is an attempt to relate protein requirements to optimum performance, which I take it is what we are really after. The question is optimum performance: What is the level at which we will get the best returns?

Sources of Calories

Could I perhaps add to this list a little? There are other factors which we have to consider. First of all, we have to consider the source and type of calories, and the utilization of dietary proteins is tied to the number of calories available, and these, of course, can come from two sources other than the protein itself. They can come from carbohydrates or fats.

When you change the amount of fat or carbohydrate in the diet, you do get changes in nitrogen balance. These in the rat are very transient; in man they go on a little longer, but in neither case do they appear to be, eventually, of any importance, and the conclusion is that within the normal limits of food composition the source of the calories is not going to be an important factor in utilization of the dietary protein.

CALLOWAY: If we go outside the normal food limits and put the carbohydrates at zero, then what would you say?

MUNRO: Well, we have the Eskimos to answer that—not completely, but under their primitive dietary conditions they had very little carbohydrate.

CALLOWAY: And quite a lot of protein.

MUNRO: Yes. The amount of protein in that case was about 300 gm. a day, which is two-and-a-half times the normal intake—perhaps three times.

Under these conditions you will eventually get back to nitrogen equilibrium, although there is an initial loss of nitrogen when you transfer the subject from the normal diet to the carbohydrate-free diet. But the evidence, which is not very extensive in man, shows that this is probably the answer, that you do get back to equilibrium even in the absence of carbohydrate. The data come from Silwer's 1937 work in Scandinavia.[18]

CALLOWAY: At what protein intake?

MUNRO: At three levels of protein intake—very low, intermediate, and quite considerable.

WARD: Can men function normally on 300 gm. of protein a day?

MUNRO: One or two explorers have adopted the Eskimo habit, particularly the Canadian Stefansson, who lived for one year, along with a colleague called Anderson, on this particular type of protein-fat diet. Anderson, as I recollect it, developed pneumonia during the course of this. Stefansson survived very well and claimed to be absolutely fit.[19]

SCHWEIGERT: If you are interested, they have a book called *Fat of the Land* which describes all these experiments.[20]

MAYER: Stefansson spoke with great evangelistic fervor against carbohydrates, which he thought were the source of all evil, quite undeterred by his succession of coronaries, and continued to claim that this was a very good diet, until he died.

EPSTEIN: What did he die of?

MAYER: Of a coronary, I think.

FREMONT-SMITH: At what age?

MAYER: Not very old—seventy-two, or something like that.

FREMONT-SMITH: He was old enough, though, and very active previously.

MAYER: This is the problem. We have no good long-term data on what the nature of diet does to performance, and by and large what there is in the literature is very colored by subjective influences. Chittenden felt fine on a low-protein diet; ergo, a low-protein diet is good for everybody—and so on.

TAPPEL: There have been military trials, though, of high-fat diets, using sort of a pemmican basis, mostly, I think, on the advice of Stefansson They had military men on a bivouac eating this type of diet, and I think they were out something like five days; they developed ketosis and became very tired, and they had to quit.

MAYER: There is a general agreement that on carbohydrate-free diets, at least for a while, there is a lassitude that sets in, but the people who are enthusiastic about them say that eventually it disappears.

BROBECK: Is it not the change in the diet rather than the composition that is important?

CALLOWAY: Apparently it is the metabolic mixture being utilized that governs the ketosis. The respiratory quotient of fasting subjects or those receiving diets that produce traces of acetone is about 0.75. According to the very old literature, the minimum amount of carbohydrate needed to provide a theoretical ketogenic-antiketogenic balance is given by the formula: $\frac{\text{total kcal per day} - (100 \times \text{grams of urine } N)}{50} = \text{carbohydrate}$ in gm.[21] Therefore, if the diet provides a minimum of protein (producing about 6 gm. of urinary nitrogen) and the energy requirement is 2600 kcal., then 40 grams of carbohydrate (or metabolically equivalent glycerol, triose, etc.) should either just prevent or just permit ketosis.

Very recent studies in the chicken have demonstrated that 0.7 to 1.0 part of glycerol or glucose per 10 parts of fatty acids is sufficient to correct growth depression from diets supplying 15.4 kcal./gm. of protein. Converting these values to human equivalents at the 2600 kcal. level yields a calculation of 168 gm. of dietary protein and thus according to the formula above a need for 2 gm. of carbohydrate in the presence of the 214 gm. of fatty acids needed to make up the calories, the same value as in the chicken.[22] This mixture is about the same as the composition of sirloin steak or good Cheddar cheese.

BROBECK: While we are talking about this, I am often impressed by the large amount of folklore that is around college training tables as to what is the right diet for optimal performance.

In many colleges the football players apparently are supplied with beefsteak every night and, if my information is correct, usually for lunch. There is nothing known in nutrition about the adequacy of beefsteak that suggests to me that this is going to guarantee a winning football team, and yet coaches believe absolutely in this kind of diet. I wonder if there is not some way to get into this particular situation and try to get some reliable data about what diet does to athletes.

K. SCHWARZ: Several Olympic teams have done this.

MAYER: There is a long tradition of high-protein diets which can be traced back to the fifth century BC, as a matter of fact, and what objective data there are would suggest that performance is somewhat better on a high-carbohydrate than a high-protein diet.

People forget—they get so obsessed with the fact that you get 9 calories per gram of fat but only 4 calories per gram of carbohydrate that they forget that in most sports the problem is how many liters of oxygen and how many calories can you produce per liter of oxygen?

It is the amount of oxygen which is the limiting factor, and there you are actually better off if you metabolize carbohydrates than if you metabolize fats by a factor of several percentage points. So, if anything, the theoretical data and some practical data would show that you are likely to do better in endurance sports by metabolizing carbohydrates.

MUNRO: With regard to synthetic diets involving amino acid mixtures, there is conflicting data as to whether or not the caloric needs of the subject are increased beyond those subjects consuming full protein.

First of all, the actual observations are in dispute; and, secondly, I am not at all sure that the interpretation, even if there is a real difference, is at all valid. So this should be held in mind if at a later date we come to the question of synthetic mixture feeding.

MAYER: The difference is simply enormous. Professor Rose said he had to increase by 1000 calories a day to maintain these young men he had on pure amino acids.[23]

MUNRO: I think that means that they were not in balance, because the mixture was deficient, and the extra calories will temporarily put you into balance.

FREMONT-SMITH: May I throw into the discussion: If we are really going to be concerned with optimal performance, then we must not neglect a very crucial—perhaps the most crucial—aspect of the diet, provided the rest of the diet is reasonably adequate; and that aspect of the diet is motivation.

We know from many experiments that the presence or absence of a high motivation enormously changes the performance of an individual, provided he is not in a depleted state.

So I think this is very important to be borne in mind, and, therefore, the subjective aspects, how a person feels, is going to play a dominant role, if we are measuring in terms of optimum performance.

SCHWEIGERT: That is in part what is behind this training table, I am quite sure—the prestige item and the flavor and the taste.

FREMONT-SMITH: And the general expectation from the coach and from high authorities that it is going to work is a terribly important aspect. It is the placebo effect, so-called, which is the motivation effect.

WARD: What do they feed during the game and immediately before? Carbohydrates—dextrose?

BROBECK: According to this account they get steak the morning of the game.

WARD: Are gastric difficulties more frequent with heavy meals like steak, because of tension?

MAYER: As a matter of fact, in terms of football games where you are not going to use the platoon system and you are going to use people for fairly prolonged efforts, you are better off if you feed them closer to the game, which you cannot do if you feed them a heavy fat meal, and a liquid diet is probably the way by which you can bring nutrition closest to the game without having any sort of gastric difficulty.

SCHWEIGERT: I am glad to see that at Harvard you have first-hand knowledge of this kind of thing. Very good!

CALLOWAY: Could I ask a question about the amino acid diet? Would it matter whether you had nonessential amino acids as compared to a source of nitrogen such as ammonium citrate?

MUNRO: That is a difficult one. I think the evidence suggests that ammonium citrate plus a carbohydrate source will probably suffice.

CALLOWAY: In that case you are saying that carbohydrate is essential.

MUNRO: Carbohydrate is certainly essential. There were some studies done by Geiger [24] at the University of Southern California in which he showed that under conditions of no nonessentials, he needed carbohydrate in the diet to make the nonessential amino acids in order to prevent the breakdown of the essential ones, but that is a highly artificial situation. Perhaps we should defer this until the discussion later on.

The last problem is quite a serious one. We do not know for a certainty whether people who engage continuously in heavy work—that is not people who are going into athletic training, but heavy laborers—do in fact require a higher intake than the one which is given as the standard one; or, conversely, whether people who are at rest have a lower requirement.

The evidence is very sketchy. I think Jean Mayer has some data which are of particular interest in this connection, because, as I recollect, he demonstrated that rats forced to work will still grow on the low level of protein intake, and grow better as a result of the increased calories required for the extra work. In other words, if you consume more of a poor diet because your work demands extra calories, that extra protein in the poor protein diet is used for growth, and is not diverted because of the increased caloric expenditure. This would imply that there may not be an increased protein requirement in the case of subjects undertaking fairly strenuous work.

The other factor which has not been mentioned is that on low-protein intakes there is some evidence of mental slowness. There is some suggestion that subjects become rather apathetic.

BARNES: How low? What are we really talking about in terms of the level of protein that affects mental acuity? It seems to me that these are very important questions, and we really have not come to grips with them as yet. We have not defined the type or level of performance that is important, and furthermore, we do not know whether or not one gram or half a gram of protein per kg. provides for the better performance.

MUNRO: I think this, of course, merely reveals the state of play at the moment; but there are no answers to these questions which are acceptable.

SCHWEIGERT: You have some recent work bearing right on this problem.

BARNES: Well, in a way, but our studies involve extremely low protein intakes, which we are not discussing at the moment.

MUNRO: That is what I would like to say. The evidence is positive, is it not?

MAYER: If we are dealing with space, we do not know what optimal performance means. Even though the criteria for the selection of astronauts are very rigorous from certain viewpoints, the fact is that most of those people would not have been selected as fighter pilots during World War II, because they are too old. So that the fitness that is required of the astronauts depends entirely on the type of tasks which they are asked to perform.

For example, if they are going to be sitting for a year going to Mars and coming back, probably one of the most important types of fitness is the ability to stand extraordinarily monotonous sitting in a confined space with not much stimulation, without breaking down under it—which is an entirely different type of fitness from the type of fitness that is required to be a commando.

Again I think there is a certain unreality to speaking of nutrition for optimum performance unless we know what the performance is going to be.

MUNRO: I have just one item left on the list and that is the effects of the interaction between protein intake and injury and infection.

Again, areas of ignorance are more obvious than areas of knowledge, but after serious injury—that is, fracture of the leg or some other accident; and it is possible that these could take place—the subject does lose an appreciable amount of body protein which has to be replaced during convalescence, and this makes a demand on protein requirements.

Secondly, there is a relationship between susceptibility to infection and protein level in the diet. The exact level which is protective is certainly not known. All that is claimed from a considerable literature is that this reveals a higher susceptibility to infection of subjects and animals on really low protein intakes; but what is the optimum for resistance to infection I would not care to say.

MAYER: Is it not true that the optimum varies? When we speak of resistance to infection, we may speak of susceptibility to catching the infection, withstanding the infection, and recovery from the infection. In the last stage there is certainly no doubt that there is an increase needed, and the higher the better.

I do not think the evidence is quite so good on catching the infection, and the relationship between protein intake and susceptibility may depend on the infectious organism nor is it quite so good on the formation of antibodies, which seems to continue even in a very enfeebled organism.

CALLOWAY: What I think comes out of this discussion is that somewhere between 40 and 300 grams of protein a day lies the desirable level.

III. THE MICRONUTRIENTS

Discussion Leader:
KLAUS SCHWARZ
Laboratory of Experimental
Metabolic Diseases
Veterans Administration Hospital
Long Beach, California

K. SCHWARZ: The subject matter of "Micronutrients" is a very complex one. Several dozen dietary components are involved, and each has its own characteristics. Clearly we need to refrain from getting too much into detail. Instead, I shall try to bring out the really essential rudimentary trends which need consideration. What are the essential considerations in terms of mechanisms, values, and aims in this field, and how do they relate to man on lengthy missions in space in a tightly closed system? Short-term missions are not under discussion here.

The material of the session will be arranged as follows: The first part will be restricted to trace elements, following which we hope to briefly discuss the vitamins. The same general considerations pertain to both areas. We have the questions of requirement, its variation with the overall situation of the organism or with specific types of stress, supply, function, and interrelationships with other specific dietary constituents.

Emphasis will be on:

(1) The equilibrium-states which are of great importance not only for optimal amino acid nutrition but also for trace element supplementation and optimal vitamin supply.

(2) The question of tolerance, i.e., the relation of requirement to toxicity. This issue is most important in the trace element field but applies also to amino acids and vitamins. In the vitamin field, however, tolerance is not much of a problem, except for the case of vitamin D.

The interplay between food intake and deficiency or sufficiency of the diet has been discussed elsewhere in this symposium. This relation is of great importance with respect to each of the essential amino acids, and each of the vitamins with the exception of vitamins D, E, and K. Anyone who has worked with diets deficient in just one of these essential constituents will know that animals will almost immediately, or very soon after they begin to be maintained on such a regimen, reduce food intake greatly. Secondary deficiencies frequently develop. If this should happen in a closed system in space, a vicious cycle may be generated.

Following the discussion of essential dietary constituents, especially the trace elements, we shall deal with peroxidation, food stability, the question of antioxidants, and of radiation. The effect of radiation in propagating peroxidation and impairing food stability may be important in space.

Trace Elements

Until approximately 1950 six trace elements had been identified as essential: iron, iodine, copper, manganese, zinc, and cobalt (TABLE 2). In 1953 molybdenum was added to the list. The physiological roles of selenium and chromium were found within the past decade in our former laboratories at the National Institutes of Health. It seems, on the whole, as if research on unidentified nutritional factors has entered a new phase. It is drifting unavoidably towards the discovery of new trace or ultratrace element requirements. After clarification of the organic constituents, primarily amino acids and vitamins, over the past half century we are now in a position to prepare synthetic, or rather semisynthetic diets of reasonable purity. The main *organic* requirements of an experimental animal such as the rat are truly known today, with the possible exception of Factor G [25], but new, unresolved *inorganic* trace-factor requirements can be shown to exist.[26]

TABLE 2

Discovery of Trace Element Requirements

Iron	17th century	
Iodine	19th century	Chatin, A., 1850–1854.[31]
Copper	1928	Hart, E. B., H. Steenbock, J. Waddell, & C. A. Elvehjem, 1928.[32]
Manganese	1931	Kemmerer, A. R., & W. R. Todd, 1931.[33]
Zinc	1934	Todd, W. R., C. A. Elvehjem, & E. B. Hart, 1934.[34]
Cobalt	1935	Underwood, E. J., & J. F. Filmer, 1935.[35] Marston, H. R., 1935.[36] Lines, E. W., 1935.[37]
Molybdenum	1953	de Renzo, E. C., E. Kaleita, P. Heytler, J. J. Oleson, B. L. Hutchings, & J. H. Williams, 1953.[38] Richert, D. A., & W. W. Westerfeld, 1953.[39]
Selenium	1957	Schwarz, K., & C. M. Foltz, 1957.[29]
Chromium (III)	1959	Schwarz, K., & W. Mertz, 1959.[27]

I shall use chromium and selenium in this presentation to delineate the principles involved. Each serves to demonstrate certain features which may be crucial for the management of trace elements in space travel. Subsequently, I will show a simple, "Trace-element-free" system for the maintenance of laboratory animals, and present evidence for a new trace-element deficiency disease in rats maintained in this closed system on highly purified diets.

Chromium

The story of the discovery of chromium as a bioelement illustrates the following two points:

(a) A trace element deficiency may document itself in relatively minor changes detectable only by certain tests, even though the defect may be of great importance.

(b) Even diets considered to be optimal by normal standards may be deficient in a specific, essential trace factor.

The psysiological role of chromium was detected in 1959 by Walter Mertz and myself[27, 28] when we tried to identify the chemical nature of a dietary factor, the so-called glucose tolerance factor (GTF). The project grew out of our original work on dietary liver necrosis and the discovery of the biological essentiality of selenium.[29] We had found that animals on certain laboratory diets had greatly impaired glucose removal rates. Not only ordinary, semipurified casein diets, but also rations containing 30 percent Torula yeast induced the impairment after four to six weeks. The latter diets were used for the production of necrotic liver degeneration.[30] The defect in glucose assimilation was clearly due to lack of a dietary agent since it could be repaired over-night by feeding of some dietary ingredients, for instance, brewer's yeast, or liver, or by application of kidney powder extracts. The impaired glucose tolerance was the only deficiency symptom observable; we used it as an assay for the fractionation and chemical identification of the GTF. Ashing of concentrated GTF fractions showed that the factor was inorganic in nature. Trivalent chromium, Cr(III), was identified as the active ingredient. The dose level of chromium required for the cure of the impaired glucose tolerance is in the area of 10 to 20μg per 100 gm. of body weight, but much depended on the chromium compound used.

Characteristic complexes and their activity in the GTF assay are presented in TABLE 3. Very stable chromium complexes are inactive because the element is biologically unavailable. Thus, the acetylacetonate (No.1) and also (most)ethylenediamine complexes (example: No. 2) are ineffective. Good results are obtained with the oxalate and the partially hydrolyzed biguanide complex (Nos. 3 and 4). After a single application by stomach

TABLE 3

GLUCOSE TOLERANCE FACTOR-POTENCY OF CHROMIUM(III) COMPLEXES

	Dose, mg./100 gm. Body Wt.	No. of Animals	Glucose Removal Rates	
			Before Supplement	After Supplement
Chromium(III) acetylacetonate, $[Cr(C_5H_7O_2)_3]$	0.02	4	1.7 ± 0.5	1.5 ± 0.4
Bis(ethylenediamine) complex, *cis*-$[Cr(ed)_2Cl_2]Cl$	0.02	4	1.7 ± 0.4	2.3 ± 0.4
Potassium trioxalatochromium(III) $K_3[Cr(C_2O_4)_3]\cdot 3H_2O$	0.02	4	1.5 ± 0.2	3.9 ± 0.8
Bis(biguanide)chromium(III) sulfate, $[Cr(C_2N_5H_6)_2(H_2O)\cdot(OH)]SO_4$	0.02	8	2.1 ± 0.3	4.1 ± 0.6

tube these induce the reconstitution of normal removal rates of approximately 4 percent of the excess glucose per minute. It seems as if complexes of intermediate stability are most suitable.

The effective levels of chromium are physiological; the element is widespread and abundantly present in nutrients, dietary supplements, and in tissues.

Not only so-called purified diets and Torula diets, but also ordinary laboratory diets were deficient in GTF.[40] Before 1960 it was difficult to find a commercially available pelleted chow for rats which would provide sufficient levels of GTF activity. In order to obtain animals which performed normally in the glucose tolerance test we resorted to feeding of kitchen scraps. These were used as GTF-positive controls. It is past history, but worthy of observation that a well-known commercial laboratory chow has been used for over three years as the basic GTF deficient diet for our studies. The producers of laboratory chow, of course, have adjusted their diets in the meanwhile to a sufficient GTF level. However, it is a reasonable assumption that until approximately 1962 much basic research on glucose utilization has been done with rats and other species which were marginal, if not deficient with respect to this agent.

Impaired glucose tolerance is often the very first and most sensitive sign of incipient diabetes. In older rats on GTF deficient Torula diets, Schröder and Mertz have recently detected a truly diabetic condition.[41] The exact correlation between diabetes and chromium is under study. There is hope that in some, but probably not in very many cases of human diabetes chromium could be used therapeutically.[42]

The mode of action of chromium is not as yet clearly understood. It appears as if the element were a cofactor of insulin. In *in vitro* systems with tissues, for instance, the epidydimal fat body technique, chromium greatly enhances glucose uptake.[43] It will do so, however, only in the presence of small amounts of insulin. The levels of chromium needed are exceedingly small. The effective concentrations are below 0.001 mg. for 100 gm. of adipose tissue in 3 ml. of medium. It is conceivable that chromium is related to insulin binding.[44] Mertz and collaborators have recently shown that during the utilization of a glucose load, the chromium levels in blood rise and fall simultaneously with the elevation of glucose and insulin in the blood stream.[45] The normal blood chromiun level is in the vicinity of 0.03 μg per ml of serum.[46]

Interrelationships: Competition and Substitution

Chromium is bound in serum by the β-lipoprotein fraction, as shown by electrophoresis after supplementation of trivalent, radioactive ^{51}Cr. Studies by Leon Hopkins and myself have led to the conclusion that chromium is physiologically transported by transferrin, which travels in the β-lipoprotein fraction.[47] The so-called "free iron binding capacity" in blood, i.e., the transferrin not occupied by iron, thus determines the ability to transport not only iron, but also chromium. Chromium competes with iron for transferrin.

Please note that this is an example of a truly competitive interrelationship between two essential trace elements. It is caused by the affinity of the two elements to the same binding site (see below). Both are positive trivalent ions, and both have a strong tendency to form hexavalent coordination complexes. The amount of iron normally present in serum is much greater than that of chromium. It would be interesting to study chromium metabolism under conditions where all the available transferrin is taken up by iron, i.e., in hemosiderosis and hemochromatosis. Most patients with hemochromatosis develop a diabetic condition within one to two years after onset of the disease. It is my suspicion that this may be related to the fact that the excess iron blocks the effective utilization of chromium in such cases.

The effect of chromium is highly specific. We tested 47 other elements for GTF activity in the course of studies which led to the identification of chromium as the active principle. Only manganese produced occasionally positive results. It is well known that, *in vitro*, many trace elements which are cofactors for specific enzymes can effectively substitute for each other. Manganese is a typical example. Enzymes which require manganese can operate *in vitro* with other, similar trace elements. This, however, does not mean that the *dietary* requirement for manganese could be replaced by any other element. To my knowledge there is not a single example of true substitution—in the nutritional sense—known in the trace element field. This high specificity in the whole animal may be related to special mechanisms required for absorption, transport in the blood stream, and membrane permeability at cell walls and subcellular structures. These barriers must be overcome by any element before it can be effective at the site of action. In the whole animal, in contrast to *in vitro* enzyme systems, antagonism, rather than positive trace-element substitution or synergism, is the customary finding.

Selectivity and specificity of trace-element requirements in nutrition may go one step further: Chromium occurs mainly in positive trivalent and hexavalent ionic form. Hexavalent chromium ions were found to be inactive in the GTF assay. Only the trivalent form of chromium is effective. With respect to recycling of biosubstances in a space capsule, the question of the eventual state of oxidation or reduction of an element may therefore deserve attention.

The behavior of most essential trace elements can be understood only in terms of coordination-complex chemistry.[48] At the bottom of trace-element substitution and competition lies the fact, of course, that elements of the same kind are similar in their physicochemical properties and exhibit similar affinities to any binding site in their environment. The behavior of the series of transition metals, for example, towards complexing agents is in principle the same, except that different members of the series have quantitatively different affinities to one and the same set of ligands.

Seven of the nine trace elements presently identified as essential for the mammalian organism are metals. Their ions have the capability and the very strong tendency to form coordination complexes. Depending on the element, they will bind 2, 4, and 6 ligands (coordination—valency). Coordination bonds vary greatly in strength. In most cases they are relatively weak. However, they can be very strong and exceed the stability of covalent C–C bond in organic molecules. An infinite variety of coordination compounds is in existence, owing to several circumstances:

(a) As ligands in such compounds, a very large number of substances may function. Theoretically, a trivalent chromium ion, which is hexavalent with respect to coordination (example: $[Cr^{3+}(H_2O_6)]^{3-}$ is in equilibrium with any substance in its surroundings which contains O, N, S, P, double bonds, or numerous other entities which could be used as ligands. This leads to a situation where a metal ion, like Cr(III), would be in a state of equilibrium with practically every organic compound present in a cell or in blood. For each of the positions in a complex, the stability constant may be different.

(b) If two binding sites which may function as ligands are part of the same molecule, as for example in EDTA or protein, the phenomemon of chelation occurs. In chelation not only the afffinity of the individual ligands, but the structural and spatial details of the connecting molecules add to the stability of the complex.

(c) Two other phenomena, hydrolysis and olation, add further variety to the chemistry of coordination complexes. Hydrolysis consists of the splitting of a water molecule; the OH ion stays as ligand in the complex, while the H ion is released into solution. Olation consists of the formation of –O– bridges between two or more of the complexing metal ions. Vast and rather inert coordination molecules can be formed in this fashion. These become biologically ineffective because the organism cannot release the trace metal from them. A typical example is chromic oxide; it is so inert that it is used as an indigestible marker in feeding experiments.

The mechanism which I have outlined makes it understandable that even the best designed synthetic complexing agent is not "specific" for one element and that trace elements of similar character compete with each other. Nature is far superior to the organic chemist in designing chelating agents for trace metals. The structural properties of proteins, nucleic acid, and also possibly polysaccharides offer ideal possibilities for the construction of sites of attachment which would have a perfect fit with respect to use of the "hole" for the atom, and the exact position and distance of specific ligands from the central metal ion. Zinc in the enzyme carbonic anhydrase, for instance, is bound so tightly that until very recently the experts were unable to get it out without destruction of the protein.

The actual condition in a solution containing a coordinating metal ion results from the establishment of an equilibrium situation determined by many stability constants, on one hand, and the speed with which the individual equilibria are established, on the other hand. Some of the interactions between metal ions and ligands occur practically instantaneously while other equilibria establish themselves very slowly.

Competition for binding sites readily explains why certain trace metals have antagonistic properties in biological systems. Pronounced nutritional antagonisms are well known. They occur primarily when levels of one or the other trace metal are unphysiologically high. Copper and molybdenum are in such an antagonistic balance.[49] Another example is zinc and copper.[50] Not always are the interactions limited to two elements; triangular interrelationships and even more complex situations are common. As a matter of fact, competition between only two individual elements may be the exception rather than the rule. It is quite clear that this is not limited to elements which are established as essential trace elements; it includes those which are biologically not necessary. This mechanism may account for some of the toxic effects of metals.

Competition between members of the same group occurs not only among transition metals. Another typical example is found in the group of halogens. Bromine is an antithyroid factor because it competes with iodine.[51]

Obviously, not all antagonistic relations between trace elements are based on competition for binding sites. Another mechanism of antagonistic behavior is due to the fact that some elements have a strong, direct affinity to an essential trace element. By combining with it, they may block its function. Cadmium, for instance, is well known to inhibit compounds which have reactive sulhydrl groups, especially vicinal disulfides. It is possible that the affinity of cadmium to comparable sites in tissues containing selenium is even more pronounced. It has been well established over the last few years that the injection of cadmium in small amounts will produce a serious testicular degeneration. This degeneration is very effectively prevented by small amounts of selenium.[52, 53] In this situation, not only selenium but also zinc in larger amounts is effective in preventing degenerative changes, perhaps because it forms a compound which shields the highly sensitive site of selenium from an attack by cadmium ions. Antagonistic interactions are furthermore seen among trace elements and major mineral constituents of the diet, for instance, between zinc and calcium.[54]

Selenium

A brief discussion of selenium enables us to delineate several other critical aspects of trace element physiology and toxicity. In Cr(III) deficiency only a relatively mild symptom, namely, the impairment of glucose tolerance, and the subsequent development of a diabetic condition have been observed. Selenium-responsive deficiency diseases, by contrast, encompass a wide spectrum of gross pathological changes. We know approximately 20 species which show severe, mostly fatal deficiency diseases which are preventable and often curable by selenium.[55] Most selenium deficiencies are characterized by massive degenerative changes in parenchymal organs. Liver necrosis in the rat is only a special instance of a change which involves many other tissues. In other species, other organs are the site of predeliction of pathology. Severe degenerative changes of the skeletal muscle, histologically indistinguishable from muscular dystrophy, are seen. There is also a typical degeneration of the heart muscle, associated with calcification located primarily at the endocardium. In birds, for instance chicks and turkeys, and in pigs, a pronounced exudative diathesis dominates the picture.

As a dietary agent, selenium presents a typical case for the interdependency of nutritional agents. Most selenium-responsive diseases document an intimate correlation between selenium, on the one hand, and vitamin E, on the other hand. Many of the selenium-responsive diseases are effectively prevented by vitamin E, and vice versa. This means that many of the very profound changes in the organism, previously attributed solely to vitamin E deficiency, develop only if two essential dietary factors are absent at the same time. For these diseases, I have suggested the term "ambogenous" deficiency.[56] The supply of sulfur amino acids is also critical.

Selenium may serve as a classical illustration of the difficulties which are inherent in trace-element research. For many years, the methods available for selenium analysis were quite sensitive, but not sensitive enough to determine effectively the very small amounts of the element which are biologically essential. Selenium was known only for its toxic effects. This has led to the paradoxical situation that in several countries, for example, the Netherlands, the laws require the *absence* of selenium from foods and feeds. If selenium would be truly absent nobody would be alive within a relatively brief period of time.

Selenium, in contrast to chromium, in general does not form coordination complexes. It is very similar to sulfur, and occurs either in inorganic form or in organic linkage to carbon, bound through convalent bonds. Most of us are familiar with organic sulfur chemistry and with the structure of sulfur-containing amino acids, like cystine and methionine. The organic chemistry of selenium is analogous to that of sulfur. Different selenium derivatives have vastly different potencies (TABLE 4). In natural materials of biological origin selenium is organically bound. Compounds can be found which per atom of selenium are three to five times as potent as selenite. Such organo-selenium compounds have also been obtained synthetically in the course of a cooperative study with Dr. A. Fredga of the University of Uppsala, Sweden, and our laboratory. Large numbers of selenium compounds have been synthesized and tested for Factor 3 activity against liver necrosis in the rat. Thus, chemical criteria which determine biopotency have been

TABLE 4

RELATIVE ACTIVITIES OF SELENIUM COMPOUNDS AGAINST DIETARY NECROTIC LIVER DEGENERATION

	ED_{50},* μg % Se
Factor 3	.7
Sodium selenite	2.2
Selenocystine	2.4
Benzeneseleninic acid	6.7
Selenouracil	ca.60
Phenylselenide	134
Selenium (gray modification)	Inactive (> 300)
4-Carboxybenzeneseleninic Acid	Inactive (> 300)

* The effective dose level, in μgm. per 100 gm. of diet, required for 50 percent protection.

uncovered. Many of the compounds tested were quite inactive or completely inert with respect to protection against the selenium-responsive deficiency disease. Many others were approximately as active as inorganic selenite, which may indicate that the selenium atom is liberated in intermediary metabolism and then utilized for the formation of the effective selenium derivative which presumably is catalytically active somewhere as an enzymatic cofactor. Only a few substances were found to be more potent.*

Toxicity and Tolerance

The biological tolerances for established trace elements are very different from element to element. In a few cases, for instance zinc and chromium, there seems to be very little toxicity, if any at all. Trivalent chromium is tolerated so well that one cannot determine the therapeutic index. In other cases the ratio between the effective required dose and the minimum chronic toxic dose is relatively small. Selenium serves as the typical example in this case. Toxicity of selenium in relatively small amounts is paralleled by its positive physiological potency at levels which are even smaller. The therapeutic index for most selenium compounds is in the area of 1:100. Four μgm. of selenite-selenium per 100 gm. of diet will prevent fatal liver necrosis in rats, while 300 to 400 μgm. per 100 gm. of diet shows slight, but distinct toxic influence if applied over any period of time. While the lower, physiological level promotes growth in several species, the latter level of selenium has an inhibitory effect.

The toxic levels of individual trace elements are ill defined, in spite of very thorough studies on some of them. The toxicity of various forms or compounds in which trace element might occur may be very different. Hence, it is often scientifically inaccurate to speak of the toxicity of an element, for example, of "selenium" or "lead." Especially selenium can occur in a wide spectrum of different chemical compounds which show greatly divergent toxicity, concomitant with greatly different biological potency. However, potency and toxicity do not parallel each other. We have highly potent, synthetic organic compounds of selenium which can prevent liver necrosis at dose levels supplying 0.05 μgm. selenium per day per animal. These substances are much less toxic than other forms of selenium, for instance, selenite.[55]

Not only biological potency, but also toxicity of a trace element, or rather of a trace-element compound, are highly dependent on the general nutritional status and on specific constituents of the diet. Methionine, for example, exerts a strong protective effect on selenium toxicity.[57]

A review of the rather narrow tolerances for some of the essential ele-

* Unpublished results.

ments leads to the realization that there is only a very limited margin for life as we know it, especially if concentrations are plotted not in terms of gram per gram but expressed as atomic abundancies on the logarithmic scale. A rat needs 10^{12} atoms of selenium in 100 mg. of diet to be protected against liver necrosis, while 10^{14} atoms are toxic. If, on the other hand, we reduce the protective level from 10^{12} to 10^{11} atoms the animal will die from an acute selenium deficiency. It is a miracle that life, depending on the right concentration of so many potentially toxic constituents, is feasible at all. Maybe this is putting the cart before the horse in that living systems may adapt themselves over many generations to environmental conditions much more extreme than those we know.

This, however, would be small consolation for man in space who is more or less suddenly confronted with unphysiological amounts of toxic trace elements in his immediate environment. I hope it has become clear from the above considerations that we need to monitor in space travel not only the nutritionally important bioelements, but also many other trace elements because of their potential harmfulness.

The analytical problems encountered are considerable, to say it conservatively. They are, of course, somewhat less acute if we test for toxic levels. Determination of the physiological levels in food or various parts of the food chain in a satellite would be quite difficult indeed. Great progress has been made in the field of trace analysis over the past few years. Radioactivation analysis, atomic absorption spectroscopy, x-ray emission fluoroscopy, mass spectroscopy, and other techniques are available for this purpose. Each of these methods lends itself to the determination of exceedingly small levels of certain elements, but not of others. None of them could be used as a solitary method to solve the analytical problems encountered. However, the development of suitable small-package instruments may be feasible. I understand that neutron-activation analysis is being used for the determination of elements on the surface of the moon.

The exact balance between all components is much more important in the area of the trace elements than in that of the vitamins. The competitive interrelationships between trace elements in biology and nutrition make it mandatory that we arrive at an exact definition of the optimum equilibrium of all elements involved. This will require much basic research. It is to be hoped that we may arrive at a system similar to the recently developed optimal amino acid mixtures. One of the main handicaps in defining an optimal trace-element equilibrium is that we have not yet identified all the elements which are required.

Unidentified Essential Trace Elements

Certain criteria can be applied in defining essentiality of a trace element for the mammalian organism. The most important and conclusive issue would be, of course, that a deficiency disease occurs in the absence of the element and that the deficiency is specifically prevented or cured by supplementation of the element (in suitable form) at *physiological dose levels.* The amounts which prevent the disease should be like those ordinarily found in blood, tissues, and nutrients.

Potentially essential trace elements may be characterized by a number of properties which may help in distinguishing them from those which are inessential. Workers in the field believe that an essential trace element should be present in the newborn and possibly excreted in the milk; it should be normally found in the organism and in tissues; it should not be accumulated easily to levels which are toxic; in other words, the organism should have a homeostatic mechanism for the maintenace of relatively constant levels of the element. The element should also be present in physiological levels in the average diet. Most of these postulates are self-explanatory. There are several pretenders for essentiality if these criteria are applied. The best known are arsenic, germanium, nickel, titanium, vanadium, and fluoride.

Some elements found *in vitro* in very small levels are thought to be present purely as contaminants because of their similarity to main body constituents. Strontium and barium, for instance, are considered to be concomitant to calcium in the organism. I could be wrong, but it is my feeling that in the organism nothing really accompanies anything else accidentally, except in more or less ubiquitously present amounts. Purity, from the point of trace dimensions, is a relative term: Very small amounts of each of the obviously existing elements are actually present everywhere. Exclusion of the essentiality of a trace element is exceedingly difficult, if not impossible. We come to a philosophical point: One cannot categorically exclude any element from being essential, except by stating that it is not essential *at a certain level.* This level is determined by the limitations of our analytical methods. Another consideration which could be used, but which may not necessarily hold true, is that there should be at least one atom of an essential element per cell. When calculating the numbers of atoms of selenium per cell, we find that there are approximately 20,000 atoms of selenium per cell in the rat. At the moment this seems to be at the lower limit of atomic concentration of essential agents in living tissue, as far as I know.

A Controlled Environment for Trace Element Deficiencies *

Having indentified selenium and chromium as trace elements with biological functions, I decided several years ago to set up a novel, systematic approach to new trace-element-deficiency diseases and requirements. Use was made of two developments which have occurred over the past decade:

* These investigations have in part been supported by USPHS Grant AM-08669.

ultraclean room techniques and germ-free incubator systems, on the one hand, were combined with highly purified diets based entirely on L-amino acids, on the other hand. Both of these approaches were modified somewhat to suit our purposes. We devised an improved amino acid ration. In the course of preliminary trials with conventional animals on these amino acid diets, we incidentally discovered a new *organic* dietary agent different from all the substances hitherto known to be required. This agent, Factor G, seems to be necessary for optimal growth of rats not only on purified amino acid diets, but also on other rations.[25]

The incubator (FIGURE 2) devised in our group by Dr. J. Cecil Smith is a modified version of the Trexler incubator for germ-free animals. It is constructed in such a way that there is no metal, no glass, and no rubber. Plastic is used throughout. The air is filtered through fiber glass. Each one of the incubators carries five cages with five animals each.

Rats maintained on our purified, optimal amino acid ration (TABLE 5) on the outside in conventional metal cages with glass water bottles and china food cups will grow. They appear fairly normal. Animals on the same diet inside the incubator system will develop a severe pathological condition within one to three weeks (FIGURE 3). The deficiency documents itself by lack of growth, seborrhea, shaggy fur, and loss of hair leading to complete alopecia. The deficiency can lead to death after three to six weeks. No

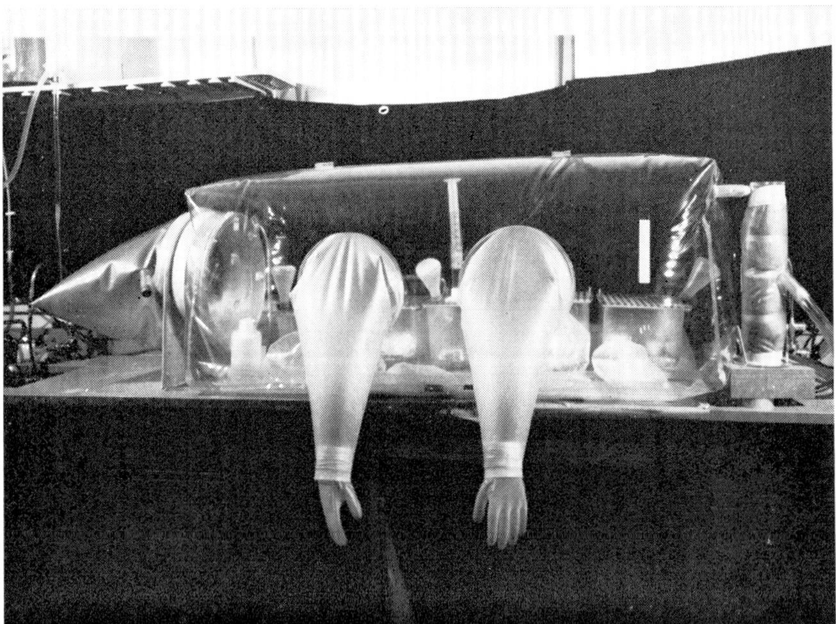

FIGURE 2. Incubator system for trace element controlled environment.

TABLE 5

COMPOSITION OF AMINO ACID DIET

Amino Acid Mixture *	17.7
Sucrose	61.2
Lard C	10
Wesson Oil	5
H.M.W. Salts	2
Salt Supplement	3
Trace Supplement Mixture †	0.1
Vitamins	1
$NaHCO_3$	1.5
Cellulose (Whatman)	2

* Composition in gm./kg. of diet: Arginine HCl, 13.0; histidine HCl, 7.0; isoleucine, 10.0; leucine, 15.0; lysine HCl, 16.0; methionine, 8.0; phenylalanine, 10.0; threonine, 8.0; tryptophan, 3.0; valine, 10.0; alanine, 4.0; aspartic acid, 3.0; cystine, 3.0; glutamic acid, 40.0; glycine, 5.0; proline, 5.0; serine, 5.0; tyrosine, 6.0; asparagine, 6.0.

† Supplying 2 mg. Zn, 0.2 mg. Mo, and 0.5 mg. Co per 100 gm. of diet.

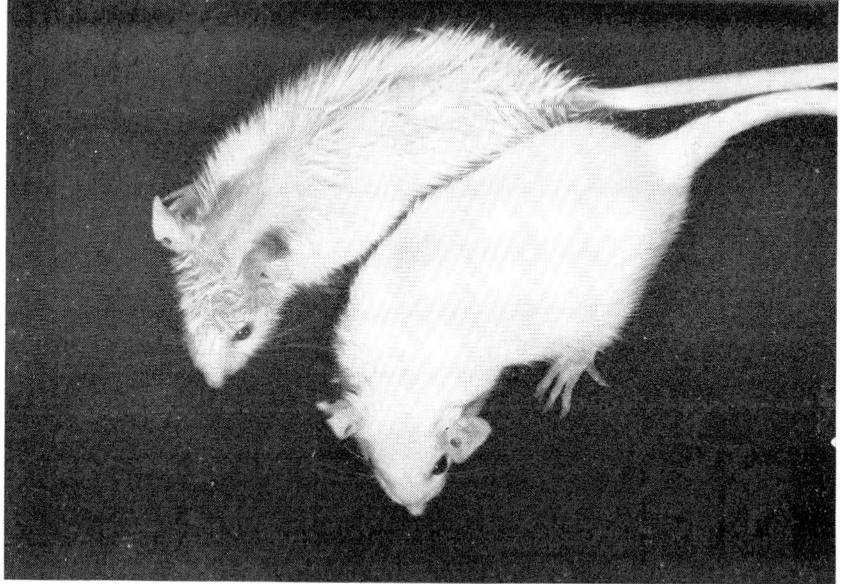

FIGURE 3. Unidentified trace element deficiency. *Left animal:* outside control, kept under conventional conditions on purified diet. *Right animal:* maintained for 20 days on the same diet in the trace element-free environment system.

specific gross pathology has been observed other than the skin condition. Animals inside the incubator on laboratory chow will perform very well indeed. They are just as good as, if not better than those on the outside.

Supplementation of 5 gm. of yeast, or other sources of essential biological factors to the amino acid diet will prevent the deficiency which develops inside in the trace-element controlled system. The same, or nearly the same, effect is seen with the ashes of yeast.

We discovered the new trace-element deficiency several years ago. Since then we have seen one failure in the course of these studies, caused by break-through of dust through the air filter. Our laboratory is in an area which is climatically very privileged. It is close to the ocean, the prevailing winds come from the west, and the climatic situation is usually described as "naturally airconditioned." However, several times each year we will have what is called the Santa Ana: a hot, dry, intense wind, coming from the desert, and carrying much dust. If the Santa Ana blows we seem to have problems with our experiments.

We have been intensely interested in identifying the trace element or elements which are missing in our system. To the superficial observer this may seem to be an easy task since there is only a limited number of elements in the universe. The complexities of the problem are illustrated by one of several episodes which have kept us occupied over the past years. For a while we thought that silicon was involved. Our incubator system is silicon-free, in contrast to the conventional method of maintaining animals. Additions of large amounts of silicon compounds, i.e. 10 to 100 mg./100 gm. of diet, produced a remarkable, positive response. However, when the amount of silicon was decreased to physiological levels, which are in the area of 5 to 30 mcg per gm. of tissue or nutrient, no effect was seen. Analysis of our purified diet showed that there was approximately 500 μgm. of silicon per gm. Part of the element was found in the amino acid mixture, and part in the salts.

Only 11 elements account for the bulk of living matter (FIGURE 4). There are nine others which are established as physiologically essential trace elements. Fifteen elements are very unlikely to be involved as essential to life: Six inert gases, two elements which have been obtained only in synthetic form, and seven which are too radioactive to be of any account in biology. This leaves us with 47 elements which are possible pretenders to trace-element function. Twenty-four of these could be taken under special consideration because they fulfill, at least in part, the conditions which have been outlined above for potential essentiality. Elimination of any one of these 24 is not easy because of the relative impurity of even the best chemicals available. Conclusive identification of the new, active element can be achieved with the help of suitable analytical methods.

The striking effect of confining animals to an isolated, very clean environ-

Trace Elements for the Mammalian Organism

established (boxed) — possible — under special consideration — unlikely (struck through)

Ia	IIa	IIIb	IVb	Vb	VIb	VIIb	VIII	VIII	VIII	Ib	IIb	IIIa	IVa	Va	VIa	VIIa	0
H																	He
Li	Be											B	C	N	O	F	Ne
Na	Mg											Al	Si	P	S	Cl	Ar
K	Ca	Sc	Ti	V	Cr	Mn	Fe	Co	Ni	Cu	Zn	Ga	Ge	As	Se	Br	Kr
Rb	Sr	Y	Zr	Nb	Mo	Tc	Ru	Rh	Pd	Ag	Cd	In	Sn	Sb	Te	I	Xe
Cs	Ba	La	Hf	Ta	W	Re	Os	Ir	Pt	Au	Hg	Tl	Pb	Bi	Po	At	Rn
Fr	Ra	Ac	Th	Pa	U												

14 Rare Earth Elements

Ce Pr Nd Pm Sm Eu Gd Tb Dy Ho Er Tm Yb Lu

FIGURE 4. The established, possible, and potential trace elements for the mammalian organism.

ment, combined with maintenance on a rather special, purified diet may have important implications for space travel, especially if one considers that man in space may be maintained on a closed, cycling, regenerative food chain.

FREMONT-SMITH: To ask a question in a somewhat philosophical vein, since life has been associated with the ocean and with water, is it reasonable to suppose that anything that was dissolved in the ocean has not been made use of in evolution in one form or another? Is there any element that you would say we could exclude, and say absolutely surely that this is not necessary in any way in biological processes or in human processes?

Gold, for instance—can we say for sure that we know that gold plays no role?

K. SCHWARZ: Gold is a very fine one. We thought some time ago we had a biological effect of gold in our relatively advanced experimentation, and I would have loved to have shown that gold is necessary for life, but—

FREMONT-SMITH: You could not make it?

K. SCHWARZ: Well, it may still come out eventually.

FREMONT-SMITH: You have not excluded it yet? Exclusion is more difficult, is it not?

K. SCHWARZ: Exclusion is much more difficult.

MAYER: Some time ago there was a lot of research in nutrition going on on antithyroid factors. People had run out of obvious dietary deficiency experiments, so they started experimenting with diet in "stress." One of the items tried was to speed up the metabolism by feeding dessicated thyroid, to see if one could create new deficiency under such conditions; and, lo and behold, certain natural materials, hitherto unnecessary, became essential, if you added thyroid to a purified diet.

K. SCHWARZ: This in part at least was chemically clarified and it turned out to be bromine—bromide. I do not think much of this has ever been published.

BARNES: This work was published. I was one of the collaborators in this study of bromide in nutrition.[58, 59]

Investigators who have been putting desiccated thyroid in diets and looking for various growth factors that may conteract the effect of the thyroid seem to have been involved with a blockage of absorption of the thyroid hormone from the gut. In other words, these growth factors were merely blocking the absorption of thyroid hormone.

K. SCHWARZ: I see. Then we go on from bromide to fluoride.

MAYER: There appears to be a growing body of evidence that fluoride is useful not only for the formation of good teeth but also for the formation of solid bones, and that there is a lot of epidemiological evidence that hip fractures and osteoporosis are far less prevalent in areas that have always been highly fluoridated naturally than in areas where the fluoride content is naturally low.

In our department Dr. Bernstein has experimented with the effect of fluoride in osteoporosis; he gave very large doses—50 mg., even 100 mg. a day—over a period of many months. This appears to be the one method of treatment that would actually keep calcium in osteoporotic bones, and it seems to have no ill effect that anybody can detect on the subjects. Apparently you can get mottled teeth with very high levels of fluoride while the teeth are being formed, but in the adult you do not get this effect.

Whether this would be useful in a situation where there is possibly a lot of calcium loss—in the astronauts—is something perhaps worth studying. But we are speaking there of more than trace amounts. We are speaking, really, of using it as a pharmacodynamic agent, rather than as a nutritional agent.

BROWN: There has been an attempt to prepare fluoride-free diets, which is chemically quite a feat, and I do not happen to know the outcome of these studies. Does anyone know?

BARNES: I know something about this. The first attempt to prepare a fluoride-free diet was made by Jesse McClendon, who raised just a very few rats on diets which were composed of natural food materials which had been grown by hydroponics with fluoride-free water, which gave him his fluoride-free diet.[60]

More recently, Maurer and Day [61] fed a low-fluoride diet to rats. Their results led to the claim that fluoride is not required by the rat. In McClendon's studies where he had a very low fluoride contnet in the diet, teeth became so soft that they fell out, and the animals could not eat, and eventually died. In the McClendon study, natural cereal grains were fed that he had raised in his own home, and he did not have sufficient quantities so that he could feed a large number of animals, and he did not include appropriate controls. He has given a possible explanation for the differences in his and Maurer and Day's results.[62]

POLLARD: This is one of the great difficulties—appropriate control. One of my colleagues, Dr. Morris Wagner,[63, 64] has been working on dental caries for over 10 years. Our germ-free rats do not develop dental caries unless they are fed a high-sugar diet and are exposed to a specific microorganism—for instance, *Streptococcus faecalis*. If you take out one of these, caries does not develop; that is, germ-free rats on *S. faecalis*—on low-sugar diets do not develop dental caries, and rats on a high-sugar diet without *S. faecalis* do not develop dental caries, but when you put them all together they do.

If fluorides are involved here, is the combination of streptococci and the high-sugar diet involved in fluoride metabolism? I do not know, but this problem of controls is something that people have to take into much more serious consideration than in the past. I am sure that people have recognized the necessity for controls in the past, but perhaps they had no mechanism by which to attain them.

Hazards Due to the Space Craft

TAPPEL: I think Dr. K. Schwarz has brought up a very important question of the complexing of these metals, which you can readily visualize as removing metals from any closed system.

For example, ferrochrome is an iron pigment which would make the iron unavailable; what if there were ferrochrome formation in the microorganisms of any closed ecological system? There are many things that will complex zinc and take it out, so I think you have hit upon a very important consideration.

REYNOLDS: This could be critical if, in a really closed recycling system, a particular trace element were sequestered in some unusable form, and therefore continually disappearing from the system.

KRAUSS: Could I ask a question which reflects somewhat the reverse of your concern that there may be insufficient trace elements.

In recycled systems in closed ecologies, one assumes that there may be microorganisms of some sort supplying some portion of man's nutrition. In such recycled systems is it likely that toxic levels of trace metals might be reached? Are any of the trace metals that are normally required at some stage of metabolism or another likely to become toxic due to a high requirement or high rate of absorption by the food organism?

Certainly you can introduce enough, but there are things like iron and copper and manganese, and so forth, which, if supplied to some other organism which in turn provides food, might indeed reach toxic levels.

MUNRO: Would this not also be coupled with chemical purification procedures like ion exchange which are liable to upset predictions?

K. SCHWARZ: My feeling is that if we upset the trace element balance and come into the toxic level, we would be more likely to do this from the engineering system than from anything else.

Mr. Arnoldi, would you want to comment on what trace elements at the moment may be most likely to be released by the system and to what trace elements the astronauts may be exposed?

ARNOLDI: I might guess the answer if we were talking about specific systems, but when we are talking generalities the field is a little too broad.

I can not conceive of any general problem. The closest to it—and this is almost a point of personal curiosity—is the question whether lithium compounds in particular are undesirable, desirable, or innocuous trace elements. Lithium compounds are common to a number of atmospheric control systems. Lithium hydroxide is used as a CO_2 control, and a certain amount of dust that absolutely has to get through into the cabin is probably ingested by breathing.

In the further future there is a possibility of CO_2 decomposition on the basis of fused salts, in which lithium compounds will be a major part. Certain vapors may escape, although part of the engineering problem is to prevent this, but there will inevitably be some trace levels of lithium compounds—halides, probably—in the atmosphere.

This is the only case where I can think of some kind of obvious interaction between the nutrition problem and the mechanical problem, so far as chemical constituents of the atmosphere are concerned.

CALLOWAY: Until you start recycling water, perhaps.

ARNOLDI: I think the water can be delivered at any degree of purity you want. We can deliver right now water reclaimed from urine at levels comparable to double distilled water.

CALLOWAY: If you take all the minerals out—

ARNOLDI: Some of them you may want to put back.

CALLOWAY: There is a separation problem!

ARNOLDI: It is easier to do the whole job. I think I answered your question by asking another question, but I would be interested in what relation lithium bears to normal metabolic processes.

EPSTEIN: Lithium is highly toxic in the rat.

GUSTAFSSON: But it has been used recently by psychiatrists for the treatment of patients in the manic phase of manicdepressive psychosis.

FREMONT-SMITH: Does it work?

GUSTAFSSON: It alleviates the manic symptoms in a few days.

EPSTEIN: Well, the rat shows a very interesting response.[65] He will initially accept lithium chloride as a substance equally palatable with sodium chloride, but after the toxic symptoms develop, he will avoid lithium salts and sodium salts, and the toxicity will develop certainly within a day of exposure, and can be fatal.

MAYER: In other words, the rat can not distinguish between sodium and lithium, and he avoids both?

EPSTEIN: That is my recollection, yes.

ARNOLDI: I am not suggesting that any large amount of lithium would be released, and whatever did get released would be in the form of compounds carried through, probably, as microparticles in the atmosphere, which presumably could be removed by suitable filtration, but the question in my mind is: How extreme is the need here?

I think perhaps your question was directed as to whether we inevitably needed to contaminate the atmosphere by other materials by any recycling process, and I think the answer to that is: No, we do not need to contaminate anything. The problem is what are we willing to pay—what do we have to pay—in order to accomplish whatever ends are desirable.

K. SCHWARZ: My question is: Where are the dangers, and where are the dangers if one of the systems breaks down—leaks, for instance?

REYNOLDS: It almost sounds like if one is really aiming toward a completely enclosed system, you would have to have it continually monitored.

K. SCHWARZ: You would need some safeguards somewhere. You would need analytical methods, and in some areas these are difficult to come by.

MUNRO: It would seem from what has been discussed just now that there are possible new deficiency diseases that might be produced by the purification of water and by recycling in the course of travel. Have any experiments been done on animals on earth with the type of recycling procedures which are envisaged with a possible view to picking up such deficiencies?

REYNOLDS: Not for long periods, certainly—not for long enough periods to—

SCHWEIGERT: How long is that? Days?

BROWN: You know this literature. Who has done a completely closed system for more than a few hours?

WARD: No one. All experiments to date have had material input in one form or another, such as oxygen, food, water, etc.

BROWN: In other words, there have been absolutely no such experiment?

WARD: That is correct. I do not believe we have any information and that is one of the big problems.

MAYER: The experiments have not been done. All that can be said is that if we have a complete food chain which is working, it is probable that the trace elements indispensable to all protoplasm will be supplied. The postulate appears to be that once you have a food chain that works, it is unlikely that it would be deficient in a basic mineral element, unless there is a differential requirement in minerals between mammalians and—other organisms.

K. SCHWARZ: We have certainly trace element requirements in plants which are very different from those in mammalian systems.

KRAUSS: These have been very precisely worked out for the algae.

POLLARD: Could you define a closed system for me that would satisfy the requirements of such an experiment?

JENKINS: Experiments with goldfish and algae in closed containers have been carried on for very long periods of time—I do not know how long, but some of these have been sealed for long periods of time, and this is a completely closed ecological system.

BROWN: A balanced aquarium, in other words; but there is no evidence that these are really in a steady state.

RAHN: If you put algae and man together, as far as I can see there is no guarantee that that particular combination will truly go into a steady state. You might by accident hit it, but you would have to find out, would you not? You cannot a priori say that if you run a mouse in an algae system, even for half a year, maybe, that you have reached a steady, closed system.

REYNOLDS: I think you could almost say right now that it is certain that you will not get it from that simple a system.

TAPPEL: Oh, yes but you could hope to keep minerals in reasonable balance by cycling through a more conventional food source like a chicken.

CALLOWAY: And I think if you put a chicken in it, it will not help too much either. You are complicating your system, and I do not think you have achieved a great deal, because it introduces another area of unknowns.

Oxidation and Antioxidants

SCHEIGERT: Could you give some insight as to whether the problems are different, relatively more complex or less complex, with respect to other features of space travel versus our normal nutrition on earth? Do you envision any new problems? We can always raise the question, but do you have any conceptual feeling or data which would suggest—say, for example, that the presence of 30 percent equivalent oxygen partial pressure in the atmosphere * influences the chromium situation?

TAPPEL: There are certain oxidant problems which anyone in a harsh environment faces, and maybe some of the oxidant problems are being faced by everybody in everyday life.

TABLE 6 tries to categorize a few of these. We discussed oxygen poisoning. This usually would occur in atmospheres rich in oxygen. The biggest problem in terms of cellular damage is probably a hemolytic episode. This has not been studied in very great detail, and there is very little literature available, I think, on oxygen poisoning, at the physiological and biochemical level.

The reactive compounds are presumed to be free radicals from peroxidation of polyunsaturated lipids. In other words, the mechanism of the hemolytic episode is fairly well established as being a peroxidation of polyunsaturated lipids of the red blood cell membrane, and this is why it breaks down. This can be protected against to some extent by antioxidants. A vitamin E-deficient person would be very liable to oxidant toxicity.

From ionizing radiation of solar flares we are protected on earth by the van Allen belt; but if you get outside of that there is a significant dose of radiation. The amount might be 10 to 1000 rad.

JENKINS: In the van Allen belt you will be exposed to a high amount of radiation—

TAPPEL: As you pass through.

JENKINS: Or if you stay in it; but outside of it there would be very little, except during solar flares, which are hard to predict.

SCHWEIGERT: That is something I would like to get clarified. Within the capsule is there enhanced radiation exposure? And if so, how much?

WARD: We had a 3^+ solar flare in 1960 during the flight of Discoverer 17. Our experiment received from 16 to 33 rads during 50 hours of fllight.

POLLARD: How high up?

WARD: Discoverer 17 was in an elliptical orbit with an apogee of about 550 nautical miles and perigee of about 100 nautical miles.

REYNOLDS: I might point out that this was below the radiation belt, so you were not getting the full dose of the flare. If you had been outside the van Allen radiation belt of an interplanetary mission, you would have gotten a dose several orders of magnitude larger.

---

* The combination of $\frac{1}{3}$ atmospheric pressure and 100% oxygen yields a partial pressure of oxygen comparable to about 33% oxygen in earth atmosphere (ASTP). Ed.

TABLE 6

FREE RADICALS AND PEROXIDES IN *in Vivo* CELLULAR DAMAGE

Condition	Cellular Damage	Reactive Compounds	Protectors
Oxygen poisoning	?	O_2; free radicals and peroxides probable	Lipid antioxidants and sulfhydryl compounds
Ionizing radiation	Nuclear and widespread	·OH, ·OOH, HOOH; secondarily organic peroxides	Mainly sulfhydryl compounds
Organic peroxides	Similar to vitamin E deficiency	ROOH	Ascorbic acid, very few tested
Vitamin E deficiency	Membrane; widespread metabolic derangement	ROO·; decomposing hydroperoxides ROOH $\rightarrow$ RO· + ·OH	Mainly vitamin E and lipid antioxidants; secondarily sulfur amino acids

JENKINS: It might be of interest to point out that in the Russian flights, up to about five days, the maximum dose that any cosmonaut received was 45 millirads.

TAPPEL: Well, radiation, in any case, is known only to be damaging, and the damage at the cellular level is both nuclear and cytoplasmic, and in the biochemical sense it comes from free radicals formed mainly from water, and so the radiation damage is indirect in a sense. The free radicals then react with the cellular constituents.

The only known protectors are sulfhydryl compounds, but the amount of protection you can get is very limited—a factor of three, namely—so you really have to resort to shielding for any protection.

Organic peroxides in the environment, of course, are harmful. Smog contains peroxyacetyl nitrate as one of its main damaging components. Organic peroxides can develop from peroxidation of olefinic compounds and so peroxides are general atmospheric contaminants.

I do not think we have to deal with vitamin E deficiency, except to say that we would not want to expose anyone who is vitamin E deficient or even vitamin E marginal to harsh conditions.

There the cellular damage is also of a similar type, usually a peroxidative damage.

The following equation tries to give a current idea about one mechanism for the aging processes; that being the reaction of oxygen with polyunsaturated fats to produce, first of all, free radicals which can damage like radiation; and these free-radical reactions lead to polymers and pigments as found in aged animals.

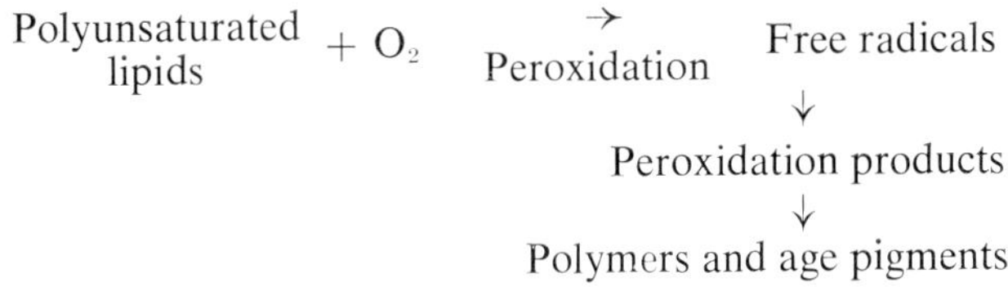

I bring this out to indicate that the peroxidation reaction may be a very basic deteriorative reaction in all biology. It is highly exothermic. It occurs widely in nature, and the damage is presumably cumulative because of free radical reaction.

TABLE 7 compares this irradiation of proteins with the lipid peroxidation reaction, and it gives more or less a biochemical comparison, to indicate that the two are the same. A comparison is given of some of the properties known for aging and age pigments. I will just point out the important properties without going into detail.

First of all, there are free-radical intermediates in both radiation and peroxidizing lipids—the yields of damage are quite similar. Of course, protein

TABLE 7

PEROXIDIZING-LIPID PROTEIN REACTION COMPARED TO PROTEIN RADIATION AND AGE PIGMENT

Property	Peroxidizing-Lipid Protein Reaction	Radiation of Proteins	Age Pigments and Aging
Free-radical intermediates	ROO·; decomposing peroxides, ROOH → RO· + ·OH	From water, H·, ·OH, ·OOH	Free radical theory of aging
Yields of protein and enzyme damage	0.004–0.02 molecule protein insolubilized per peroxy radical	0.05–0.5 molecule protein damaged per free radical pair	
Labile amino acids of cytochrome *c*	Histidine > serine > proline > arginine > methionine > cystine	Methionine > histidine > cystine > phenylalanine > serine	
Inhibitors and protectors	Lipid antioxidants including vitamin E, Se, and S amino acids	Mainly —SH compounds	Radiation inhibitors and lipid antioxidants under specific conditions
Composition	Complex of peroxidized-lipid and damaged protein; like lipofuscin	Damaged protein	Lipofuscin-complex of protein and lipid (partly peroxidized)
Solubility of polymeric part	Insoluble in HF	Protein polymerizes	Insoluble in HF
Crosslinking of protein	Protein crosslinked and polymerized		Crosslinked protein theory of aging

is only one molecule that you might consider, but it forms an interesting biochemical model.

The usual type of amino acids that are labile are methionine and histidine. These are also labile to other deteriorative reactions such as those in food processing. In fact, methionine is probably the most labile amino acid that there is. That is one reason why we have to be very careful in food processing not to damage methionine.

BARNES: Why do you say that? What kind of food processing destroys methionine?

TAPPEL: A browning reaction would, to some extent, although it is not the most labile there. Oxidative processes would.

BARNES: Would not heat destroy cystine long before it destroys methionine?

TAPPEL: Yes, but methionine is usually the more limiting.

BARNES: Methionine might be said to be more limiting if you grouped the sulfur-containing amino acids together since methionine can substitute for cystine. I do not know whether this would be necessarily true if you consider cystine as an essential amino acid in its own right, because heat destroys cystine long before methionine.

TAPPEL: Yes, and browning would destroy histidine and lysine before methionine.

SCHWEIGERT: As measured biologically (in the rat), lysine will show the greatest sensitivity to heat, but methionine is also sensitive, and, surprisingly tryptophan is not.

BARNES: Perhaps lysine is first, but you say methionine also, and I question whether this is accurate. I believe it is cystine that is really destroyed, but since you can replace cystine with methionine, everybody thinks of methionine as the amino acid that becomes limiting.

SCHWEIGERT: In these particular experiments cystine was added in a liberal excess, but that still does not answer the question unequivocally. We would be better off to say sulfur amino acids, irrespective of whether it came from cystine or methionine.

K. SCHWARZ: If we look at peroxidation reactions specifically, I think methionine does become the most vulnerable, do you not?

TAPPEL: It is the most sensitive to radiation and peroxidation damage.

POLLARD: What do you feel would be the protective action of methionine or cysteamine against radiation damage?

TAPPEL: Well, I think primarily it is the reaction $RSH + HO\cdot \rightarrow RS\cdot$, of the sulfhydryl compound with a free radical like the hydroxyl radical, and this forms an RS-free radical, and then these can usually chain transfer so that, for example, if you had two of them they could easily be oxidized to cystine in this type of reaction.

In other words, it is a competitive reaction with the free radical, preventing the free radical from hitting some labile biological constituent.

K. SCHWARZ: It is what I think you would call free radical scavenging.

POLLARD: On the other hand, could you say that since the sulfur-containing compounds are so sensitive to irradiation that you are supplementing the reserve that the animal has?

TAPPEL: Well, the animal has a natural protection against oxidants and radiation, like the glutathione group, and this can be supplemented to some extent by external—

POLLARD: Has this reaction actually been demonstrated?

TAPPEL: Yes. Of course, this kind of reaction is widely known for biochemical systems, and in intact animals I would say the result are in accord with that type of reaction.

SCHWEIGERT: For perspective, is it your conclusion also that the levels of radiation that any food component in this space travel system would receive would be limited by man's tolerance to the radiation field—and therefore, those levels are so low that they really would not affect significantly any sulfhydryl oxidation in any food component that might be in the system?

TAPPEL: I would say by orders of magnitude of ten to the fourth or more.

BARNES: Dr. Tappel, would you extend your theory of aging to say that the space traveler who is going out for many years should cut down on his linoleic acid intake?

TAPPEL: No, because I think the nutritional requirement of polyunsaturated fatty acids is primarily for building blocks for membranes, and so forth and we need a balanced amount of these, but there is apparently an oxidative deterioration of these lipids. You cannot do without them, and you are possibly damaged because of their presence, but this is a compromise that is necessary. We are aiming for the optimum, to get the best biological membranes for the operation of the body, but if we overdo it—that is, if we get too much polyunsaturated lipid and overcome the antioxidant balance, then we can get into a great deal of trouble, and of course this is the case of the vitamin E-deficient animal. You can destroy its antioxidant balance.

MAYER: What you have said is that you have to be sure to have enough antioxidants. You have not said that it is bad to have more linoleic acid, because you are going to be deficient in antioxidants.

TAPPEL: That is right.

BARNES: If you are going to consume more linoleic acid, you must take more alpha-tocopherol.

MAYER: Which is also found in corn oil?

BARNES: Not always. Corn oil can be fairly rancid or oxidized, which would destroy tocopherols.

CALLOWAY: It is high in delta-and gamma-tocopherol, but not alpha. These are effective *in vitro* but not *in vivo*, against oxidation. Cottonseed oil has a better balance of polyunsaturated fatty acids and alpha-tocopherol.

TAPPEL: I think the greatest difficulty would come if a person tried to load up on polyunsaturated lipids—even from a plant source. He could get an antioxidant imbalance, because the absorption of the fat would be very good, but the absorption of the vitamin E would lag behind.

CALLOWAY: What level of plasma tocopherol would concern you in men subjected to atmosphere enriched with oxygen?

TAPPEL: I am afraid I do not know for sure.

FENN: But would you say your astronaut should use less than 30 percent oxygen in order to prevent aging?

TAPPEL: Not necessarily.

FENN: You have mentioned oxygen poisoning presumably because you think the oxygen is going to be a little high, and would represent something of a threat.

TAPPEL: I think you would not want to go to 40 percent.

FENN: I think the chances are that anything over 21 percent will be a little bit toxic. There is no cutoff point. I know it is in some of the lower animals. Anything over 21 percent—30 percent—shortens their life, and it might very well shorten the life of a man. It is a reasonable possibility.

SCHWEIGERT: Could I ask why it is 30 + percent oxygen? There must be a reason.

LIVINGSTON: I think I could offer something and I would be glad to have it corrected by any of the NASA people. When the Mercury program was first discussed, two days after NASA was formed, on October 16, 1958, the engineers did not know at that time what shape vehicle, its size or its atmosphere. The supposition was that it would have a normal atmosphere. Sometime between that date and January, 1959, there was a decision, because of weight limtiations on structural adequacy of the Mercury configuration, that they would have to design the capsule wall too heavily in order to accommodate a full atmosphere differential with space vacuum. In the meanwhile there had been discussions about the nitrogen problem in relation to the possibility of explosive decompression. Max Fager,* who was providing background information to the Life Sciences Committee at that time, explained that they decided to go to a third of an atmosphere, quite arbitrarily, but that they were satisfied with a 100 per cent oxygen

* Maxime A. Fager: Assistant Director for Engineering and Development, National Aeronautics and Space Administration, Manned Spacecraft, Houston, Texas.

atmosphere, being assured that at 5 p.s.i. that would be practically equivalent to sea level oxygen partial pressures.

It was initally an engineering decision, not dictated by physiological considerations.

BROWN: We are assuming that the decision was primarily a physiological one, and since we seem to have eliminated that reasonable possibility, then it is presumably just an arbitrary one—but I do not think it is.

The higher the total pressure, the easier it is for the engeineers to design cooling systems. The higher the pressure, the smaller the motor has to be to provide heat transfer by conduction. So there is an advantage in having the pressure high.

However, full atmosphere, 15 p.s.i., is in excess of what the capsule turned out to be designed for, and they had to go down to something about 10 or 11. But you are working against these two extremes, one a cooling problem and the other a physiological problem.

So I think this is really a compromise, and the engineer does have a point. He wants the pressure to be as high as possible for cooling purposes. If you had used a mixed, two-gas system, you could have had normal atmospheric oxygen plus another gas making up the difference, but the complications with the two-gas system were presumed to be beyond the capability of the engineers at the time. Also, the second gas could lead to compression problems. So I think there really was some sense to it. It was not strictly arbitrary.

K. SCHWARZ: Is the oxygen pressure *within the tissues,* under the conditions which are in use in space craft, normal, or is it elevated?

RAHN: For my money nobody has ever measured the tissue pressure, but the best way of thinking of it, I think, is: What does the arterial blood provide the tissues with? And that we know, and that is approximately 50 mm. higher in the Gemini atmosphere than it is right here in this room.

This is my personal view, now: This 50 mm. added to blood which is already completely saturated with oxygen is of no account.

BROBECK: What is the mixed venous oxygen, PO_2?

RAHN: You can calculate it. It is going to be 1 millimeter higher. When you breathe 100 percent oxygen in this room, mixed venous oxygen tension rises 11 mm.; that is all.

BROBECK: So that the tissues are not going to be that much different.

MAYER: You said that that small difference does not matter, but is it not essentially what produces retrolental fibroplasia in newborn infants who are incubated? So at least under those conditions—

RAHN: Well, when you go up a little bit higher, there is a gray zone which Dr. Fenn was talking about. For his money, every astronaut is being poisoned by oxygen, because he has set the limit at 21 percent.

FENN: Yes, a little bit—I mean, just theoretically. You can never prove it, but I think anything over 21 percent probably has some physiological effect, even though it is only 50 mm.

But it is very little. I do not think it is of any great importance. If you go up to one atmosphere, then of course it is important. Then you get retrolental fibroplasia—in infants, that is; not in adults.

TAPPEL: In the adult you primarily worry about hemolysis of the red blood cells.

FENN: I do not think you worry about that primarily though. The first thing you will get is convulsions. You do not care so much what happens to your red cells.

The onset of convulsions has nothing to do with the red cells. This is something that happens in the brain. High oxygen pressures have been shown to diminish the concentration of gamma-aminobutyric acid,[66] which is an inhibitor. In its absence it may be that all the signs in the central nervous system are "go" and the result is the development of convulsions.

Another possibility is that in high oxygen you break into the oxidative chain at some point further down toward the substrate, so that you bypass points where ATP is formed. Thus, less ATP is formed with the same amount of oxygen, and this may cause convulsions or produce difficulties.

This may happen because of free radicals, but the real cause of oxygen poisoning directly is not the free radicals; it is something that they may do, like oxidizing something further down in the chain or damaging some enzyme, or coenzyme like lipoic acid,[67] or something of that sort. It diverts the metabolism to a new channel, and then either you do not get the same amount of ATP, or some reaction goes without energy, or some peroxides accumulate.

TAPPEL: It is very likely that a damaging event is the formation of the free radical and its subsequent reactivity, because it takes a very, very minute amount of this to cause the equivalent of ionizing radiation lethality.

So if you put it in terms of comparative amounts, you would have to have very, very little free radical formed in the body from, say, lipid peroxidation, which is one of the most labile sources, to be equivalent in lethality to ionizing radiation.

FENN: That is all right. You have to show what the free radicals do in order to produce oxygen poisoning or damage.

CALLOWAY: One thing is to decrease sulfhydryls in the proteins lining the surface of the lung, which would—or could, at least, theoretically—change the surface-active properties. This could be one of the reasons for lung damage experienced in pure oxygen atmospheres.

K. SCHWARZ: Lipid peroxides have been obtained and studied. Their toxic effects are primarily on the central nervous system, and those levels which you can use to kill an animal are exceedingly small. A few micrograms could kill a chick.

REYNOLDS: There is evidence that decreased oxygen tension in mammals results in a decrease in radiation sensitivity. I am not sure whether it is also true that an increased amount—

CALLOWAY: It is.

K. SCHWARZ: How much would this 50 mm. excess oxygen tension mean in terms of a hyperbaric situation? Would it be true that it would take a very small increase of air pressure to obtain a physiologic situation comparable to this 50 mm. excess oxygen? The question, furthermore, would be whether this would constitute a strain on the organism or not.

RAHN: On scuba, for example? For every 100 mm. total pressure I get 20 mm. more oxygen, so I have to raise the pressure to 200 mm. above atmospheric to give you approximately 50 mm. of oxygen.

FENN: That's about 10 foot depth.

K. SCHWARZ: I am not a scuba diver, you see. I had hoped someone might have some comments concerning this problem of oxygen tension as it relates to just plain physiological situations.

CALLOWAY: If you are worried about an oxygen hazard, could you just saturate people with alpha-tocopherol? Would there be any harm in any level of alpha-tocopherol?

TAPPEL: Maybe we can see that in TABLE 8. I have tabulated the antioxidants that man has had experience with.

Actually, there should be an optimum amount of alpha-tocopherol. Experience has shown that you cannot protect by just increasing the alpha-tocopherol infinitely. You cannot protect against radiation. You cannot

TABLE 8

ANTIOXIDANTS AND FREE RADICAL SCAVENGERS

1. Lipid antioxygenic compounds active in vitamin E-deficient animals.
   Vitamin E, especially α-tocopherol
   Trace element selenium
   Sulfur amino acids
   Synthetic antioxidants—Dihydroethoxy Triethylquinoline, Diphenylphenylene Diamine (DPPD), Butylated Hydroxytoluene (BHT).
2. Water-soluble antioxidants of animals.
   Ascorbic acid
   Glutathione and sulfhydryl proteins
3. Radiation protectors.
   Cysteamine
   Aminoethylisothiuronium bromide·HBr (AET)
   2-Mercaptoethylamine·HCl (MEA)
   Cysteine
   Glutathione

get a great increase in protection against oxygen toxicity or peroxide toxicity by vitamin E alone; but protection might be increased by using other anti-oxidants. For example, you want to be sure that ascorbic and sulfhydryl compounds are up, so that you would have a good amount of glutathione.

It might be useful in the human dietary to consider some of the synthetic anti-oxidants that have been used in chicken mash, for example, although these present their own problems as additives. And then there is the possibility of using radiation protectors, but except for cystine and glutathione, of course, these also have a level of toxicity, so that to get protection you might have to take some risk.

So, I think, except for the conventional thing which all nutritionists would suggest—that is, adequate vitamin E, adequate ascorbic acid, adequate sulfhydryl compounds—the rest of it is sort of an unknown.

WARD: I may have missed it in the discussion, but what is the maximum partial pressure of oxygen at one atmosphere total pressure that an animal can survive in and do well?

RAHN: This experiment is difficult to perform. At 1 atmosphere O_2 mammals live 3–5 days. As the O_2 is reduced to 50 percent they may live for weeks and then as one approaches the normal O_2 pressure of 0.21 atm. the animal lives its standard life time. Therefore, it is difficult to predict how much the life span is reduced by only raising the O_2 pressure by 5 percent of an atmosphere. It is difficult to do experiments on survival times at higher than normal oxygen pressures, because they take too much time, unless you go to high values like 50, 60, 70 percent oxygen.

BROWN: There must be some statistical data on the lifetime of man as a function of where he lives.

FENN: I think there are too many other factors, when you go up to altitude, social factors, and all kinds of things, and I do not think the available data would help us very much.

ARNOLDI: There is one point on increased oxygen pressure, and that is the experiment several years back at the Air Crew Equipment Laboratory in Philadelphia, where five men were confined in a chamber for one week at 400 mm. of pure oxygen, and it had no untoward effects that I am aware of.[68]

FENN: That does not say that it would not have had an effect on their life span if they had stayed there. This is an impossible experiment to do.

SCHWEIGERT: At least it is relatively insensitive to testing at that level.

MAYER: There are studies on Denver and Johannesburg both are a mile high—and there is no noticeable shortening of the life spans, so perhaps you are better off on the lower side than on the higher side, if you have to take a chance.

REYNOLDS: I think there is a noticeable decrease in life span at altitude.

LIVINGSTON: I have always heard it attributed to radiation increase at altitude, rather than oxygen tension differences.

FENN: It is much more likely that it is something besides the oxygen.

BROWN: How can you separate these? Maybe it is lower gravity.

K. SCHWARZ: Dr. Schweigert, would you like to comment at this juncture on the problems of peroxidation and food stability, specifically with reference to the situation of space travel?

SCHWEIGERT: I think I might start out with a generalization. In my own self-education here, I have not seen any striking condition that has been proposed which would markedly alter the problems we have with food stability—of constituents here on earth.

To expand that a bit, the unsaturated fats—polyunsaturated fatty acids, to be specific—are susceptible to autooxidation through chain-reaction mechanisms that Dr. Tappel has referred to. They normally occur more rapidly at elevated temperatures than they do at lower temperatures, and hence rancidity from oxidative reactions is retarded by low temperature, and that is, of course, the fundamental basis we use in storage of foods at low temperature. There are also microbiological and other reasons why we store at low temperature.

There are oxidation products associated with such chain reactions which are very deleterious to foods besides the relatively reduced acceptability due to rancidity. (Although even this is variable among people and cultures, and we have individuals who prefer rancid foods, we should remember, although certainly they would be in the minority in the United States, I would think.)

These deleterious reactions are associated with loss of vitamin E, or the tocopherol which was referred to; and of vitamin A, or the vitamin A activity from carotene and related vitamin A precursors. There is also a loss of certain of the other vitamins that are susceptible to oxidative reactions.

One of the key factors in the rate and extent of such oxidation is the presence of catalysts in complex food systems, such as iron, or iron in a coordinated form, such as the red pigment in meat, myoglobin.

I could give you one exception, just for curiosity, to the effect of temperature, and that is that certain meats, such as bacon, become rancid more rapidly frozen than they do unfrozen, and this seems to disobey all laws of chemical reaction. The presumed explanation, however, is that the solubility of oxygen is really greater in the frozen food by oxygen diffusion than it is just above freezing.

However, I would like to stress that, while we know a considerable amount about the mechanisms of oxidation and the effects of antioxidants, in model food lipid systems—in other words, a purified fat with an oxidant, given temperature, et cetera—in a food or complex biological system, the mechanisms defy simple clarification.

For example, certain of the antioxidants Dr. Tappel listed are very effective in a purified lipid system such as lard or margarine. They may be very ineffective in a mixed food system, while another antioxidant will be relatively more effective. That tells you that the interrelation of prooxidants, chelating agents which may have an influence on the rate of oxidation—the whole physical state, the amount of moisture present, are all involved almost to the degree that a red-blooded scientist would not even start such a problem.

The polyunsaturated fatty acids are much more susceptible to oxidation in certain types of lipids than in others. In the neutral fats, which, as you know, are composed of glycerol and simple fatty acids—those fatty acids are relatively less susceptible to oxidation than if they are in the form of a phospholipid, which has a phosphonitrogen base component in the molecule.

In heat treatment of foods we are concerned about thermal degradative changes in lipids. "Overheated fats" is a phrase you will hear. A generalization would be that the normal heat treatment that fats receive in food handling and food systems provides only minor toxicological problems. A few scientists may not agree with that, in the deep-fat frying of potato chips or french fried potatoes in certain restaurants for umpteen usages, but in general I do not believe this is a significant problem, even though experimentally one can produce some thermal degradation products—polymers, which are highly toxic to animals.

On an overall basis, I came with a great deal of interest to see what unique problems there would be with these foods in space. Assuming packaging competencies, sources of foods that I am familiar with, the usual processing know-how that we have, I see no major problems on nutrient retention within practical limits. I would be much more concerned with the acceptability of those foods in terms of flavor, texture, color, in relation to motivation of the individual himself.

I also would add that any more highly dense calorie sources than our normal foods, and the 20 percent or so variation in protein requirements mentioned this morning, would seem to be an area of greater fruitfulness than [is a search for] some artificial calorie substrates.

K. SCHWARZ: I would think that the deep frying of foods for space flights is in the far distance, and we do not need to worry about that for the moment, but I would like to point out that peroxidation is actually the result of antagonistic effects.

The prooxidative effect is not just due to oxygen in the food or in the mixture you are investigating. There are many catalysts for peroxidation—or prooxidation. Iron is one. Many of the trace elements we have been talking about in the first half hour of our afternoon session will have a very strong prooxidative effect. Not just that: The joke is, really, that many of the so-called natural antioxidants will have a prooxidative effect under certain conditions, and I think we have to *investigate* very carefully the stability of these foods under the proper conditions before jumping to the conclusion that they may be stable. There is no easy solution to these problems. The idea we just could charge everything with natural or synthetic antioxidants is certainly too simple and may be quite dangerous.

Cabin Temperature

LIVINGSTON: I would like to ask Dr. Schweigert about the advantages of a cooler environment. By changing from, say, 70 to 50° F. is there a considerable extension of time before rancidity occurs?

SCHWEIGERT: In general, the lower the temperature, the more stable the food is.

TAPPEL: Well, perhaps if we spoke about freeze-dried foods, which have been investigated intensively by the Quartermaster Corps—they have stability in excess of one year of 100° Fahrenheit.[69] But these are protected by inert atmosphere. In fact, that is necessary; otherwise, they would not last a week because of oxidative rancidity.

This would extrapolate to something like six or seven years at room temperature, so presumably one could go on a flight for several years and carry enough freeze-dried food of good quality.

LIVINGSTON: This question is of special interest; there is not likely to be a lot of refrigeration aboard. Last year we heard about three major problems relating to astronaut well-being:

One was the problem of cardiovascular reflexes—the question of how the astronauts would be able to cope with weightlessness in flight, modest gravitation on a planet, acceleration on return to the earth, and acceleration on landing on earth. A second problem was that of decalcification in the weightless situation. A third problem was water balance.

Each of these three problems is affected in the right direction—that is, in the direction of being advantageous to the astronaut in terms of fitness—if he lived in a cooler environment. I am interested to learn additionally that one of the major nutrition problems—that of rancidity of food products—is also affected in the right direction by having a cooler environment.

This really becomes a footnote to last year's conference. I thought it probable that NASA, with its magnificent facilities at Houston, would have begun to approach an answer to this question by testing on the ground the potentially beneficial influences and reasonable limits of temperature reduction in the capsule.

The specific answer as to how much temperature drop you should have in order to get how much advantage in each of these three physiological areas and in the area of food storage needs to be tested empirically. I do not believe it can be extrapolated from existing experiments; but since in each case a cooler environment is advantageous and since knowledgeable people like Per Scholander and Hammel say that the degree of advantage is likely to be appreciable, I think it might be an important contribution from these Conferences to suggest that this be tested carefully.

Whether it would be most advantageous to have a steady low environmental temperature or a steady low environmental temperature with intermittent periods of still lower temperature is a question that might also be desirable to test.

BROBECK: Dr. Livingston, what is the temperature in the capsules as they have been used?

LIVINGSTON: They have aimed for something around 80 degrees, have they not?

REYNOLDS: Seventy-eight.

BROBECK: And is this attained by heating or by cooling?

REYNOLDS: It has been by solar heating plus a water boiler.

SCHWEIGERT: We could add the generalization that the quality or value of foods is certainly improved, if any change occurs as to lower temperatures. There will be exceptions to that, but that is the generality.

K. SCHWARZ: But it would lead to increased food requirements.

MAYER: But this is only beyond the zone of thermal neutrality. It is not true within a certain range of temperature.

LIVINGSTON: Conferees estimated last year that it was not particularly disadvantageous to have metabolism boosted by a cold environment; I am glad to hear Dr. Mayer confirm that. Appetite is also affected in an advantageous direction by a relatively cool environment. Is that not correct?

BROBECK: Yes.

LIVINGSTON: So I do not know anything against lowering the environmental temperature down to some level that can be acclimatized or adjusted to; and I know of at least four or five advantages in respect to recognized problems in space travel, each of which is affected advantageously—and some quite substantially—according to data now available.

FENN: You do not want to shiver your way all the way to the moon, though, do you?

LIVINGSTON: That is right, but you do not have to do that.

BROBECK: Eighty degrees is probably too warm for optimal performance, is it not?

LIVINGSTON: I think so, and all the astronauts have complained about over-heating, before takeoff, during flight, and most especially after landing.

BROWN: Does not the reduced pressure make some difference in the effective temperature?

LIVINGSTON: It increases the water loss.

REYNOLDS: And it also decreases the heat loss.

LIVINGSTON: You are saying that when you are at a reduced pressure, it is even more important because of the lowered pressure to have a lowered environmental temperature.

BROBECK: Yes, because it is hard to get rid of the heat.

MAYER: Dr. Schweigert said he could see no special problems in food technology. I assume that we are back in the context of a situation where the flight is short enough, and—

SCHWEIGERT: I am not talking about closed systems.

MAYER: The problems become quite different if we talk about long flights, and I suppose that one of the things we ought to address ourselves to is the possibility of producing antioxidants in sufficient amounts in closed systems or self-regenerating systems. Has anybody looked into that at all?

CALLOWAY: We presume chlorella would be fairly high in tocopherol, but I do not know.

TAPPEL: Many plant sources are very good.

K. SCHWARZ: Some of the algae are very highly unsaturated in their fats.

SCHWEIGERT: They are also quite low in fat.

FENN: I think it is about time to adjourn. Do you have a few last words for us?

Vitamins and Variation

SCHWARZ: It is deplorable that we have had no time to say anything about vitamins. Astronauts cannot survive without them. Let me at least submit a few basic aspects which deserve your consideration.

The first one, of course, is that of vitamin supply. In the report of the Conference on Nutrition in Space and Related Waste Problems,[1] I found a statement that it was decided to use the recommended vitamin allowances of the National Research Council. To me this is a most dangerous situation and one about which we ought to think twice. Vitamin requirements are highly variable not only from person to person, but also from one situation to another. They depend on the degree of activity, the amount of stress, the type of stress encountered, and many other variables. I would suggest that we try to calculate what would be an optimal supply, particularly since there is not much of an additional weight load to be added.

MAYER: Plus the fact that there are great variations in requirements, there is even greater variation, apparently, in the ability of the organism to hang onto the store.

Vitamin A deficiency is fairly common if you look at the world at large. It may be the second or third cause of blindness in the world. Yet in trying to produce vitamin A deficiency in hitherto well-fed subjects in Britain, it took 18 months before there were any signs clearly ascribable to vitamin A deficiency and not even in all individuals.

MUNRO : Ten out of 16 showed reduction in blood of vitamin A and deterioration in night vision. None showed epithelial changes, and none, of course, showed corneal degeneration compatible with incipient blindness.

MAYER: And the same thing is true in vitamin C. One of the striking findings about vitamin C is that typically Spanish or Portuguese navigators would leave their homes with rather a large crew and three or four ships, and would come back with 20 percent of their complement, everybody else having died of scurvy, but the 20 percent they had still going were apparently doing well with no visible source of ascorbic acid in the process demonstrating a tremendous variation in the ability of adult human subjects to hang onto their stores of almost anything.

K. SCHWARZ: Of course, I think this again points to the fact that you should screen your astronauts for abnormal requirements, before you put them on the trip.

The second item of basic importance which I like to mention is that a deficiency of a single, essential dietary factor will lead to a negative feedback mechanism with respect to appetite. A vicious cycle can be precipitated which produces a great number of secondary nutritional and other disturbances. There is no doubt that man in space will be subject to this risk. Incidentally, what is being said here about the vitamins is also true for amino acids and for other dietary ingredients such as trace elements.

The third principle which is noteworthy is that of balance. There is a connection between the requirements of various vitamins. Vitamins have to be provided at dose levels which are balanced out against each other if serious impairments of function are to be avoided. Balance, of course, is also important in trace-element nutrition, amino acid nutrition, and in the supply of the main dietary components on the whole.

Lastly, let me point out that there are several important areas of nutrition, in the basic sense, about which we do not know very much at all. There are, for example, very strong indications that we do not know all the factors which are required. This pertains not only to the trace elements discussed above, but also to the organic components of a diet. In our laboratory, for instance, we have found that a new, unidentified factor (Factor G) is necessary for optimal growth of animals on amino acid diets.[25] It is possible that Factor G is a new vitamin. If we come from basic knowledge to knowledge on nutrition of the human species, things become much worse. We do not even know the exact requirements of the human with respect to many of the vitamins which are well established as required by mammalians, bacteria, etc. This is related to the fact that the human does not lend itself to prolonged rigorous nutritional experiments with seriously deficient diets. It would be foolish to assume that the human does not need biotin, pantothenic acid, or vitamin E just because we have not been able to demonstrate this experimentally.

IV. APPETITE, SATIETY AND FOOD ACCEPTANCE

Discussion Leaders:
JOHN R. BROBECK
Department of Physiology
University of Pennsylvania
School of Medicine
Philadelphia, Pennsylvania
and
FRANK W. HEGGENNESS
Department of Physiology
University of Rochester
School of Medicine and Dentistry
Rochester, New York

FENN: This morning's session will consider the crucial question: Will he eat it? Dr. Brobeck will lead the discussion.

BROBECK: Thank you, Dr. Fenn. What I have to say this morning was written down some years ago in a monograph on physiological problems in space exploration.[70] I should tell you that my chapter got a going over by some of the reviewers, who said I did not know what I was talking about, and I am sorry to tell you that my knowledge of this subject has not improved any in the past three years. But I have not altered my opinions.

I believe that I am here representing two different groups. Together with Jean Mayer and Al Epstein, I represent a relatively small group of investigators scattered around the world, all the way from New Delhi, through Taiwan, across this country and to Stockholm at least, and possibly going on into the U.S.S.R. This is the group of people who have been interested in the control of food *intake* by the nervous system.

However, I represent also another group [concerned with questions of food *preference* or selection]. Perhaps most of us were too young to be asked what should go into the rations that were fed men at the time of the First World War, but we are old enough to have been on the Conferences the second time around. The subject of these conferences was this: Now that we have made up all these wonderful foods, how come these ungrateful soldiers will not eat them?

Dr. Barnes and I were brought together by a mutual friend of ours, Sam

Lepkovsky, who spent about three years organizing a basic research program on food intake that had some of the most prominent names in medicine and biology in this country in it. To the best of my knowledge, the Quartermaster Corps supported basic research for about three years. From that time, so far as I know, the interest of the Quartermaster Corps' laboratory has gone more and more toward practical work, that is, food acceptance rather than fundamental study.

So far as our discussion this morning is concerned, I see this as a very simple problem, which I shall try to illustrate as follows: Let us suppose that on any March 8 a rocket was launched with a crew of some size on their way to some mission way out in space; it's now possibly the 12th of September, and these men are away out there yonder. The question is: What are we going to have for breakfast today? And for lunch and for supper?

You will know that there is no fundamental science that will tell us what these men are going to want to eat under such conditions at that time. No matter how carefully we may scrutinize the kind of studies that Dr. Epstein, Dr. Mayer and others of our friends have done, they are not going to answer this question: What are these guys going to want for breakfast on any given day, or the day after or the day before?

Food Habits, Training and Experience

So far as I can learn, there is only one kind of answer to this question. It is the answer that the Quartermaster Corps' laboratory came up with; perhaps some of you will wish to challenge the way I express it. I conclude that these men are going to want for breakfast what they had been eating before they took off. As I see this problem it is a mistake to send men on a mission of more than a few days, or maybe a few weeks, until we are able in an engineering sense, to put up a PX with them. I am confident that the Armed Forces have put these excellent markets in Taiwan and in Korea and in other remote parts of the world for a very good reason: they have found that this is the only adequate way to feed their people under these conditions.

JENKINS: What is the experience from prolonged submarine missions?

BROBECK: It is the same as the one that Dick Barnes and I were involved in during the war. The men complain about the food, and they will not eat it. I do not know a great deal about this, although some of us on the Navy Committee for reviewing Navy research in this field may—It has been one of the serious problems.

CALLOWAY: Not any more, apparently.

REYNOLDS: I do not think it is true of submarines, but the submarines, in order to take care of this problem, had different foods from the rest of the

Navy. The submarine service was the reason for the Navy going into boneless beef in large quantities. They ate essentially home-style cooking all the time on the submarines.

BROWN: I understand obesity was a problem.

REYNOLDS: That is right.

BROBECK: But there is none of this nonsense that if it is a simple diet and if the men are well-motivated and hungry enough they will eat it.

I am not suggesting that we must send along a great variety of foods, but I believe that we should send the capacity to make them. Where we were talking yesterday about the possibility of sending along a standard milk-shake mix which can be made vanilla one time, and chocolate or strawberry another time, I decided that we should aim for something more than that. We should plan to send some fundamental building material that can be served as corned beef one time, as hamburger another time, and on another occasion as beef stew.

This is not impossible; there are techniques already for converting basic proteins into fibers and for processing the fibers. If I were in charge of this program, I would go after the people that manufacture synthetic fibers, and I would ask them how to take the broth from an algae culture and spin it and knit it into a hamburger, so that I could serve it to this man when he wants a hamburger for lunch after he has been out there for about eight months.

We were also asked about the man who is ready to go into combat who does not want to eat; what can we do for this man to enable him to eat his last meal before he goes into fighting? My answer to this is very simple and straightforward, and is along the line that Dr. Mayer was talking about yesterday. It is: Forget about it. If the man is not ready nutritionally to go into battle on the morning of the battle, it is too late then to worry about it. The time to think about his nutritional state is in the three weeks before fighting, and again when he comes out, and not during the time he is actually in combat.

I suppose that for men in space this problem applies only to the blastoff and to the reentry phases. On these extended missions that we are talking about the man is going to be much more like the fellow who is stuck on a Pacific Island and is sitting out the war for two or three years without anything very exciting happening. The astronaut's requirements are going to be more like those of a man occupying a missile base than like those of a man going into combat every three weeks.

BARNES: I would like to ask you a question. For years you have been studying the factors that control voluntary food intake and you have been successful in identifying certain of them. To my knowledge, in all of this work that you have done that deals with the control of food intake, you have never become involved in questions of flavor, texture, and other similar psychological factors. Now, why is it that you set aside your knowledge of the fundamental factors involved in the control of food intake and talk about the importance of flavor and textures and things of this sort?

FREMONT-SMITH: You mean, why does he talk common sense after having been in science?

BARNES: No, sir! I will not go along with that. I am not so sure that it is common sense. I am just questioning Dr. Brobeck's view that this is the important thing to be concerned about—to be able to give the man a hamburger rather than to be able to give the man a certain nutrient intake.

BROBECK: It seems to me that there is not any basic science to be applied to this kind of feeding problem, so we have to go at it from a common-sense point of view.

The rest of our group may not share my conclusions, but if the NASA people asked me to design a diet for a man who is going to be in space for six months, these are the principles that I would use.

MAYER: I wonder if what you are saying is not really much more a matter of the psychology of being in an environment where there are very few sensory stimuli, if indeed this is the case (if you are not being talked at by Colonel "Shorty" Powers every second, or whatever is going to happen in space), because from what we know about behavior of animals and man, as deprivation becomes more prolonged, the sensory aspects of food become less important.

BROBECK: Do you mean food deprivation, or sensory deprivation?

MAYER: As food deprivation is more prolonged, the taste, texture, and so on, of food becomes less and less important. The satiety mechanism is like a brake which is slowly being released, so that inhibitions or difficulties which were very important when the animal was quite sated become less and less important as the animal becomes hungrier and hungrier.

FREMONT-SMITH: He will eat almost anything eventually.

MAYER: Obviously, this is not the situation in which we want to put the astronaut, but the fact is, if the need is there, unless the food is extraordinarily repulsive, it will be eaten, and human experience shows that this is the case.

This is not to say that they would not rather have hamburgers, but they will eat almost anything if they are hungry enough.

That is one thing. The second thing is something I have seen operate. If you put men away from their social system, away from their wives, their daughters, and in an entirely different, new situation, they will change the food habits very radically very easily.

This is, for instance, what is happening all over West Africa as men are being imported to work in harbors, in mines, in industrial enterprises, and so on. You can change their food habits with remarkable ease, and, as a matter of fact, in many cases the nutritional difficulties that we encounter are due to the fact that people have changed their traditional ways of eating very easily.

What you cannot change is the technology of cooking. If women in a given area know only how to handle foods in certain ways, and you present them with foods that they cannot cope with, then obviously you cannot change their food habits. If they do not have the implements, if they do not have the knowledge, obviously you cannot get them to prepare different foods. But this is a much different situation, and I am not at all sure that one could not have a very successful program with foods which are unfamiliar, even though it would be important from a morale viewpoint, perhaps, to give them familiar foods.

BROBECK: You spoke of this when we were talking about the K rations, where certain items were preferred and were taken out, and the soldiers threw away the rest. Now, according to the nutrition people, the rest of the stuff was what the men really needed, but they never acquired the habit of eating it.

I never ate a K ration in anger, but I tried to eat them in a laboratory—and this was the improved K ration, not the original one. The original package was good for throwing at the enemy, I was told, whereas the second one, the improved one, was supposed to be edible. Even our graduate students would not eat it.

MAYER: Nothing in the K ration was familiar; let us put it that way. But some of the items, although unfamiliar, were palatable.

MUNRO: To what extent does this fastidiousness about food vary from one person to another? In other words, could you select individuals who were more tolerant than others?

BROBECK: Yes, I think this is important. It seems to me that the easiest and most reliable way to find out what this man is going to eat in space is not to show him a cafeteria two days before he takes off and expect him to pick out what he will want, but to find out what he has been eating in the past two years. If you find a man who does not seem to be very fussy about food, who does not complain if the potatoes are burned or if they are fixed in a new way, or if the dehydrated potatoes don't taste "like Mama used to make"—if you select a man of this type, it will be much easier to feed him than a man who must have his food done in just a certain way.

This is one place where selection is entirely possible, and training as well, but I would not send a man out into space and train him there. I would spend the two years before he goes training him here, so that he will know what he is going to get. I believe that what Dr. Mayer says is right: You can persuade these men to eat a lot of odd things, but six months in space is not the time to start it; the training ought to be started before they are taking off.

Meal Frequency

MUNRO: The second point that I would like to raise is frequency of feeding in relation to rejection. Is there any relationship between the amount that has to be taken—that is, say, dividing meals into eight instead of four—and the acceptability of the ration?

BROBECK: The question you have asked leads to the most important point of all this: We need much more fundamental research on these problems in human subjects. We can tell you about frequency of feeding in laboratory animals; but about men I do not know—maybe the nutrition people know more about this than I do.

MUNRO: I have personal experience of nitrogen balance studies [71] many years ago, in which the meals were divided into either two per day or eight per day—the diet, for simplicity, was basically made of bread and butter and jam, and simple things like that—quite monotonous.

On the eight meals a day it was perfectly acceptable, because one never felt either full or empty. In fact, it was a very comfortable state of pleasant half-satiety, and I wondered whether on the basis of this single personal experience, which is, therefore, not statistically significant, rations that are rather monotonous and not too acceptable may be more easily taken in frequent small meals, than in one large, rather nauseating mass.

BROBECK: All I can suggest is that it ought to be looked into. Dr. Mayer, do you know anything about this?

MAYER: We have just completed a study of hunger and satiety sensations in a thousand men, women, and children, and the variability of people as regards just that sort of thing is very striking. People experience hunger and satiety in different ways. There are a great many things in common, but there are also a great many differences in the way in which sensations of hunger and knowledge of satiety are felt. There are differences between men and women, differences between adults and children, but the answer to your question is that it depends on people. To what extent this is an acquired phenomenon reflecting the way they have been eating over the years, and to what extent it affects individual physiology and psychology, we do not know.

The second thing which is important is to realize that in the West we are used to food that comes in chunks. We eat a steak, a lamb chop, a portion which is a large, discrete amount. We know from the British work, for instance, and others, [that in these populations] the day-by-day adjustment of food intake to energy expenditure is very poor, and it is only over a fairly long period that you achieve balance.

When you study people who eat food which comes in a much more continuous form, like people who are essentially rice eaters, where most of the calories come from rice, the day-by-day adjustment of food intake to energy expenditure is very much better.

Now, whether this is due to the fact that they are not faced with a choice between one sandwich or two sandwiches, one steak or two steaks, but just a little more rice or a little less rice, I do not know; but I think this may be important in permitting them to adjust their food intake to their energy expenditure somewhat better on a day-by-day situation.

HEGGENESS: The initial observation that led to the suggestion of feeding as well as diet composition as an important factor in the body economy was made by Tepperman, Brobeck and Long in 1943.[72] They showed that animals made hyperphagic by hypothalamic lesions and restricted to the caloric intakes of control animals, had postprandial respiratory quotients suggestive of high rates of fat synthesis. Later work by van Putten, van Bekkum and Querido [73] confirmed these findings and showed, by carcass analysis, greater fat accumulation in hyperphagic animals eating once a day. Later, Cohn,[74, 75] and others,[76] have shown that intact animals (mainly rats, without hypothalamic lesions) fed large infrequent meals accumulated more fat and less protein than control animals eating the same amount of the identical diet.

FREMONT-SMITH: Did not Tepperman and Tepperman do experiments quite a ways back in which they conditioned rats with shocks so that they were only allowed to eat at one time of the day, and when they did this, with no change in diet, the rats became extremely obese?

HEGGENESS: Tepperman, Brobeck, and Long [72] observed the high respiratory quotients in hyperphagic animals pair fed with control nonhyperphagic rats and suggested that this was due to the feeding pattern: As the animals were always hungry they ingested the food provided immediately; the control animals ate more leisurely. This observation was confirmed by Dutch workers.

FREMONT-SMITH: Do they not get obese? I thought I saw pictures of them.

BROBECK: This is the impression that has gotten into the literature, Frank, but it is not quite true. What the animals get is a very high capacity for synthesizing fat, but they do not tend to become obese. They have a different composition of the body.

HEGGENESS: They do add significantly more body fat and less protein.

MAYER: The difference is significant, but it is not a great difference. The effect on cholesterol may be much more important, but the effect on total body fat is not great.

EPSTEIN: It is the effect on lipogenesis which is common to both experiments.

BROBECK: That is right. We found it first in the hypothalamic animals where in a fed state the R. Q. was as high as 1.3. Dr. Tepperman [77] went on to show that this was not a consequence of the hypothalamic operation nor even of the obesity. He could train normal animals to have this high RQ by space-feeding them.

MUNRO: We made a few observations of corticosterone levels in the plasma of rats trained to consume fixed meals at fixed times of day, and these undoubtedly rise as a result of training. This, of course, would affect the distribution of body fats.

HEGGENESS: There have been a few studies on humans suggestive that feeding pattern may be a factor in determining blood cholesterol, the shape of the glucose tolerance curve, and urinary nitrogen excretion.[78–81]

MUNRO: It must be remembered that hormones like growth hormone respond extremely rapidly to food. For example, glucose decreases growth hormone in plasma very quickly at the same time that the insulin content rises; and these adjustments are rapid and transient.

MAYER: There are striking differences in the way people consume their calories. We not only have people in the population who have different numbers of meals and snacks, but people who eat a very large fraction of their calories in the morning, and others at lunch, and others in the evening, although most of the American population consume most of their calories at night.

BROBECK: We think that we eat three meals a day, but actually the common American custom is to eat six. These are not of uniform size, and some of them are not big enough, perhaps, to be called meals, but many people have something for breakfast, have a snack with coffee in the middle of the morning, a lunch of some size, a bit of food with coffee or tea in the afternoon, and then dinner; and it is very common to have something to eat before you go to bed.

MAYER: Considering that it is true that there are some people—a large proportion of people—who have six snacks, or three meals and three snacks —on the other hand, we have been very surprised to find out that there is a very large number of men in the United States who have only one meal a day. They eat practically nothing at breakfast and skip lunch with great regularity and have one meal, often followed by after-dinner eating, and that is their pattern.

This is not unknown in the world. I remember the experience I read of a large mine in South Africa where people customarily eat only one meal a day, a large meal after they come out of the mines, and the physiologist of the mines had the idea that people would be more efficient if they ate more often. They tried to convince the workers to eat more, and the way they did it appeared simple enough.

Those are very deep mines. People have to wait—the workers have to wait sometimes as much as an hour-and-a-half to get into the elevators that service the mines. They wait in long lines, and the idea was just to put food along the line so people could eat as they went in, and nobody ate. The one time they wanted to eat was at night, after the work was done.

We have a great many people in our society who voluntarily choose that pattern and have all the physiological or psychophysiological accompaniments, in terms of gastric hunger contractions, feelings in the head, feelings in the back of the mouth, and so on—all the various types of hunger sensations—appearing only once a day, and the posteating change of mood also appearing only once a day.

We have no basis, really, for thinking that one pattern is basically superior to another. I know that there has been work done by Clarence Cohn and others suggesting that snack-eating is better than meal-eating in terms of blood cholesterol, and so on, but it's really a relatively small effect.[82]

If we put people in an entirely different type of environment, do you think that one ought to try to conform to what has been their rhythm of eating, or do you think that ought to be changed, or could be changed, according to some of the things that Dr. Munro said?

My own feeling is that we do not know.

EPSTEIN: This change in the rat's feeding frequency, if I could just make a minor correction, is not the change to meal eating. The rat is a natural meal eater, but he eats small meals. This is a very old finding of Richter's [83] from the 1920's.

HEGGENESS: I think intermittently fed animals differ from ad libitum fed animals in that they alternate between the absorptive and postabsorptive state and that the influx of nutrients must be much larger during a finite period following feeding than that of ad libitum fed animals. Intermittently fed animals show many adaptive changes in the gastrointestinal tract.

EPSTEIN: I am only saying that the rat is a meal-taker; he is not a nibbler. This is a common misconception that I find among people who do not know rats. They are not constant nibblers. They are meal eaters.

K. SCHWARZ: Could we get the facts? When do they eat, and for how much of the time do they eat, and how many times a night do they eat?

EPSTEIN: It depends on the diet. On laboratory chow an adult rat will eat perhaps a dozen to 20 meals in a 16-hour period, beginning in the late afternoon and going into the midmorning.

K. SCHWARZ: But it would not eat during the daytime proper, would it?

EPSTEIN: Some. Very little.

BROBECK: What we are objecting to is the statement to that this is a question of meal eating versus nibbling. More correctly it is big meals versus small meals.

EPSTEIN: That is the point. You are imposing a very large one or two meals on an animal that ordinarily takes a dozen to 20 small meals.

MAYER: Migrating birds are a very curious story. They show the real function of obesity. The characteristic of being able to store enormous amounts of fat may be saving the life of an organism, including men under certain conditions. The animals that fly across the Gulf of Mexico manage to do it essentially on their fat depot, and I think something like two thirds of their body can be fat before they go off.

POLLARD: Since we are talking of patterns of eating, is there anything to be gained from studies on the Australian Aborigine, as far as his diet patterns are concerned and his ability to withstand long periods of privation?

BROBECK: There are data on this, but like many other data relating to human food intake, they are not quantitative in the sense that we have data on rats.

I talked about this with Ted Hammel [84] after he came back from his study on temperature regulation on these people. The ones he studied are essentially what Clarence Cohn would call nibblers. They are like grazing animals; they are always looking for food, and they eat it when they find it.

EPSTEIN: It is an economic necessity.

BROBECK: There really is not much food available. He described a very wide variety of materials that they use for food. Although they may go from one feast to another as far as killing an animal is concerned, most of the time they are living on berries and beetles and a lot of things that we do not eat, which they use as food sources.

MAYER: The thing is, unless you study it in detail, it is difficult to know whether you are dealing with people who actually have no hunger feelings for long periods, or whether you are dealing with people who have learned to be captains of their souls, and so that while the hunger feelings are there and just as violent, they will disregard them.

BROBECK: They show something that is odd about food intake. In their studies of temperature regulation, Howard Hammel [84] and the others found that these people will sleep with a cold sky over them and no covering, under conditions where their rectal temperature falls by a degree-and-a-half or two degrees. This is not surprising. What is surprising is that they do not wake up and go for some food—because I think any of us would certainly wake up with this fall in temperature, and most of us would wake up thinking of food.

I do not know whether it was because under the conditions of the experiment this was excluded. Under natural conditions, it is possible that they would wake up and eat in the middle of the night. But at least in the experiments that were done in the cold trucks and under the cold sky, they did not do this.

BARNES: We have a curious observation in rats, which may be of interest to you, though it is preliminary. In the course of a study of the rehabilitated rat, that had been deprived of food for the first three weeks of life and then rehabilitated for a period of eight to 12 months, we were getting into the use of operant testing procedures that involved food reinforcement.

In order to do this you have to have rats that are hungry. We did this by feeding them only one hour each day.

There were about 60 rats in this study, about 15 of which had been deprived of food for the first three weeks of life. They all lost weight when we put them on the one-hour feeding. I should add that these were Holtzman strain rats, which are known for their placid nature.

About eight of the 15 rats that were deprived of food during the first three weeks of life became very vicious and would attack and bite your hand when feeders were put in their cages or were being removed. We had to wear a heavy glove when handling the feeders in the cages of those animals that had been nutritionally deprived in early life. They appeared more highly motivated for food than the others.

Now, whether such a thing could carry over for a year in the life of a rat, I would not say for sure, but at least in the famous first experiment this is what it looks like.

BROBECK: This is interesting, because it is my impression that everyone who has taken care of animals with lateral hypothalamic lesions has been impressed with how easy they are to handle. By contrast the medial lesions, which are the animals that are getting fat, must be handled rather carefully. There are people who say they are difficult or impossible to handle.

MAYER: I think that is not strictly true, Dr. Brobeck. I think it is true if the lesion has beeen made by stereotaxic instruments, but it is not true if the lesion has been made by gold thioglucose.

BROBECK: But the gold thioglucose animals have all kinds of other lesions.

EPSTEIN: And the gold thioglucose animal is a mouse, not a rat.

BROBECK: This has become a private argument here, and I am sorry.

In the part of the brain that apparently controls food intake in a quantitative sense there is a medial system the destruction of which leads the animal to overeat and become fat. When it is stimulated, it stops feeding. Dr. Epstein has shown that it can be anesthetized and its activity is temporarily suppressed, and that the animal will overeat during this period.

FREMONT-SMITH: You mean, the area can be anesthetized?

BROBECK: That is right. The lateral hypothalamus, which lies just beside it, a millimeter away in the rat, upon destruction gives an animal that does not eat at all for a while, and eventually may recover from this aphagia, but still shows deficits of control of food intake. Upon stimulation, this area induces feeding.

Now, what we are discussing is: Is there a correlate of emotional behavior, difficulty in handling the animals, that goes along with the location of these lesions? I have said what I think is true. Everybody who has had rats with lateral lesions is impressed by how easy they are to handle. Is that not what you would say?

EPSTEIN: I used to, but I think now this is just a wider range of emotionality. You will find some very placid laterals, and you will also get some very jumpy ones.

BROBECK: We have never had those. The ones with the lateral lesions I have always found it easy to handle, and the lab boys have no trouble with them.

EPSTEIN: Whereas the medial animal is uniformly a vicious animal.

BROBECK: Well, it depends on who is handling them. I have never had trouble with them, but in general the lab men do.

MAYER: This is the result of hitting all sorts of other centers, because if you do ventromedial area lesions in the mouse, stereotaxically, you show this result, whereas if you do them by gold thioglucose, you do not.

In rats there are strains which will resist the toxicity of gold thioglucose, so—

FREMONT-SMITH: What is this?

MAYER: It is glucose linked to gold by a sulfur bridge, which is injected, and which destroys specifically certain cells of the ventromedial area, and the animal becomes very obese. And these animals are not vicious, although they are quite hyperphagic, so I do not think the two things are necessarily related. I think they are related by way of geographic overlap.

BROBECK: In cats nobody has separated the viciousness from the obesity. People who have had fat cats have always had vicious cats; but in monkeys it is the other way around, and we have a very strong impression that the first evidence that the operation is successful and that the animal will be hyperphagic and will get fat is that he has lost his fear of the people in the laboratory. He will come up to the front of the cage the morning after the operation when you come in to see how he is getting on.

Eating and Neuropsychiatric Responsiveness

BARNES: There is a lot of attention being given to food in terms of its psychological and emotional values to the individual, and to the feeding and the feeding patterns in terms of these psychological and emotional values.

Experiments that have been done with animals indicate to me that an animal performs muscularly, and perhaps intellectually, better if he is partially starved, and there are some indications that this is probably true in man also. I do not mean long periods of starvation, but if they are hungry, men might perform better.

The idea of always keeping a full belly to maintain a man in his best condition may not be true. I am not saying that this is the thing that should be done, but I think there should be some question thrown into this discussion that keeping a man emotionally happy because he has a full belly may not be the best thing for him. Furthermore, it may not be the best thing for him to provide him with hamburgers or something else that he likes to eat, just because of his emotional relationship to that food item.

BROBECK: This is the next topic that I was going to suggest we discuss, and I will summarize my impression of it by a quotation from Herman Hickman, who was a well-known after-dinner speaker and raconteur, and, incidentally, a football coach, who said: "It is the job of the coach to keep the alumni restive, but not mutinous." The object of feeding is to keep the man alert, but not mutinous.

I shall attempt to introduce this topic by reminding you of three fundamental facts about food in laboratory situations that are sometimes overlooked. The first one is: By all laboratory tests of alertness and intelligence, the bright animal is the starved animal. If you compare learning times or any kind of criteria of central nervous system performance, the animal that has been without food for 18 hours is the one that has the advantage over the one that has just been fed.

So far as I can learn, practically all studies in experimental psychology are done on fasted animals. Originally, perhaps, this came over from biology, where the development of biochemistry and the study of metabolism made it obvious that scientists had to have some baseline metabolic pattern that they could use in comparing different species of animals and different treatments. So they established the conditions of basal metabolic study as being the uniform, standard metabolic state.

Psychologists may have arrived at it independently, but the principle is well known to animal trainers. The animals that are trained for circuses and performing acts are never fed *ad libitum.* They are fed on some kind of a schedule where the feeding comes as a reward.

FREMONT-SMITH: Is this not also an element of motivation? In the normal living of an animal, if he is hungry, he is alerted to seek food; he has a real motivation to do something.

So I think one would expect this from a biological evolutionary phylogenetic and ontogenetic point of view. The animal that is hungry is going to be more eager, and one of the main jobs that an animal does is to seek food.

BROBECK: It seems to me that we are both making an interpretation.

FREMONT-SMITH: I am doing this on purpose.

BROBECK: I said the animal was brighter, and you said the animal was more highly motivated. One might say that the animal is more likely to be active. All of these are interpretations of what we see.

However, the fact is that experimental psychology is based upon the study of the hungry animal.

K. SCHWARZ: It is my understanding that intelligence is measurable and that it is different from motivation. Can you or can you not separate these issues in psychological tests?

FREMONT-SMITH: Well, he may appear to be brighter because he is motivated.

BROBECK: In the animal situation these cannot be separated.

CALLOWAY: Studies at Northwestern University, under Quartermaster support, used avoidance conditioning, which is a way of trying to separate it, for evaluating alertness at various times after feeding in the dog.[85] They found that the hungry animal was more alert to centrally located visual cues but less alert to those that were peripheral; that is, he made more mistakes in response to peripheral cues when he was hungry, but fewer mistakes with centrally located cues.

FREMONT-SMITH: What is a peripheral cue?

CALLOWAY: Using a large panel of lights, the ones that are on the outside edges.

BROBECK: I would like to make the other two points.

The second one is: Food is the oldest tranquilizer. The mother does not feed the baby because the baby is hungry. She feeds the baby because he is obnoxious.

FREMONT-SMITH: That is right, because he cries. How can you use such an interpretive statement as "obnoxious"?

BROBECK: Well, he is noisy, then. The baby is noisy, and the mother provides a tranquilizer. Food is the first tranquilizer to be used in our lives, and it is the oldest one in the history of the race. This, I think, relates to the point that Dr. Barnes made.

The third point is one that Sherrington [86] made in 1900, when he wrote his treatise on the spinal cord, for the Schäfer textbook on physiology. He said that hunger state affects the whole nervous system, when he was trying to get ahold of the same problem we are talking about. He said that in studying spinal reflexes he had discovered that if he used an animal that was just fed, and then cut the spinal cord to study the reflexes below the section, he found that the spinal reflexes were depressed.

He said that if he wished to have an animal with active reflexes, he took a well-nourished animal and starved it overnight. He then found the spinal reflexes to be the most easily demonstrable. His conclusion from this was that there must be, therefore, a spinal state of hunger.

So these are the points I wanted to make, that starved animals are the "bright" animals, that food is a tranquilizer, and that it affects all levels, apparently, of the complex nervous system.

RAHN: You used two words, a "starved" animal is a more "intelligent" animal, and then the next time you said the "brighter" animal. These are not good words. Would "alert" be a better term, which is less subjective?

BROBECK: I have been using synonyms, because there is not any precise word for it. They perform better under tests.

MAYER: I wonder to what extent, though, Dr. Brobeck, this is not reflecting our technology of testing animals. The easiest way to reward an animal for doing something is to feed him. You can also give him an animal of the opposite sex, but this requires a considerably greater—

LIVINGSTON: There are lots of ways of controlling this, Dr. Mayer. You can use punishment as well as many other kinds of motivation. You can also use secondary rewards.

BROBECK: If you want an animal to work for heat, for example, you starve him before you put him in the cold.

MAYER: The second thing is starving versus fasting, and so on. Surely it is useful to differentiate the degree. Short-term deprivation may increase alertness. Certainly long-term does not, and neither in animals nor in man is it particularly good in terms of being alert to things other then your own immediate comfort.

The third point, which may perhaps be more relevant to selection of astronauts or to their handling is this: When you work on men rather than on rats, you are struck by the fact that there are considerable differences in the way in which stress and food are related.

Now, there has been a lot of what I can only consider as mythology written by psychiatrists about the symbolic value of food. It makes good reading, but there are very few data as to what it actually represents.

What has struck us is that there are at least two kinds of people. There are the people who eat more under stress, and the people who eat less under stress or when they have tasks to perform. Now we are doing a number of determinations on these two types of people, such as circulating catecholamines, circulating insulin, and so on.

Society imposes a stress very periodically on young people in the form of examinations. It is a stress that recurs in life, and if you start looking at the evolution of food intake and weight of people at those periods, some people always gain weight during the examination periods while some people always lose weight then. Their approaches to food during those periods, and their hunger sensations, and so on, are quite different, and this is what we are interested in at present.

My feeling is that we are going to find that some people are helped to pass examinations by having eaten a good meal before they take the examination. Some people perform better during examinations when they do not eat.

At least, I would like to reserve judgment on any sort of generalization as to what we are going to find in men, in terms of reaction to stress as a function of psychological, and physiological idiosyncrasies.

To give an example of other differences in individuals, there are some people who spend less than 1 percent of the time of a meal talking about what they are eating, while for some people the time goes up to 50 percent. Surely this is an important difference. This is the sort of thing that ideally one would like to know about the people who are being sent on long missions.

LIVINGSTON: Dr. Mayer, I would like to make a hypothetical prediction, that in these two populations of people who prefer to eat, or not to eat, in relation to stress—that they would also be divided according to whether they were people who preferred to be relatively vasoconstricted or relatively vasodilated, and I think it would be possible to test this in your questionnaires with fairly simple choices. I mean, by asking whether they like cool temperatures or warm temperatures.

MAYER: I think there are differences in body types which may go along with these psychological differences. My feeling at this point is that the people who are predominantly mesomorphic would rather eat under stress, and the people who are predominately ectomorphic would rather not, but I do not know yet.

SCHWEIGERT: We need help on those two words.

MAYER: These are Sheldon's [87] classification of body types: ectomorphic, characterized by elongated extremities; mesomorphic, characterized by large bones and muscle mass; and endomorphic types, who are rounder and have, at least potentially, a lot of adipose tissue.

There are great differences in body types, for instance, in susceptibility to obesity. We find that girls who have hands which are long enough in relation to their width—to the width of the hand—never become obese; that only certain types are likely to become obese.

Now, similarly, it is highly probable that the attitudes toward food of the various types are also different.

FREMONT-SMITH: At least possible.

CALLOWAY: We have been involved in assessment of food attitudes and personality traits quite accidentally because of having to select subjects who will be able to tolerate for a long time the formula diets we use experimentally. I do not know why, but our psychologists independently rule out the same volunteers on the basis of psychological tests as we do on the basis of food questionnaires. I would like to know what characteristics we are evaluating in common. We are fairly successful in selection because our drop-out rate is remarkably low.

BROBECK: What criteria do you use on your questionnaires?

CALLOWAY: The subjects' own statements about how often they are willing to eat specified foods, preferences for flavors, tolerance to a wide variety of foods—probably most importantly, tolerance to a variety of foods, combined with willingness to eat things repetitively. I am not altogether certain which psychological tests are prognostic; personality inventories and various kinds of mood scales are administered and group interviews are conducted.

FREMONT-SMITH: I think that the point of small meals really deserves special emphasis, because nausea is certainly cumulative, and if a person is taking a very small meal and gets just a little bit nauseated at the end of it, this is one thing, but if he has got to double it, then the nausea becomes much more than double, and it might be that the food would be rejected, so that if the size of the meal could be small enough so that even if it was nauseating when stopped just before the nausea really amounted to anything, by the time the next meal came four hours later one might be ready for the same thing.

Biological Cycles

BROBECK: This leads to the question of cycles and feeding patterns. There is an article on cycles by Dr. Halberg [88] in Dr. Hardy's monograph which some of you might find interesting. To the best of my knowledge this has not been studied in human subjects on any large scale, but most of us have had the experience of becoming out of phase during extensive air travel. Anyone who has had it is likely to come to the conclusion that if he is going to go off in space, he would like to keep his customary cycle. I see no reason to change this, although there may be reasons for manipulation of the capsule where the man has to be waked up periodically.

K. SCHWARZ: Does this not suggest a very much more fundamental problem; namely, are these people capable of maintaining their diurnal cycle at all?

BROBECK: It probably does not matter whether they maintain cycles of the previous duration, because the data from men in caves and other isolation experiments are to the effect that, although it may drift a little bit, the cycle will drift with some kind of inherent rhyhm which eventually may be a few hours off. But if a crew is going around the world or off in space, with two or three men in the capsule, they will entrain one another, so they will all have the same rhythm. If the man is alone, it is not going to matter whether he is off by a few minutes or a few hours anyway.

K. SCHWARZ: From previous week's missions is there anything known about a drift in body temperature cycles?

REYNOLDS: These missions have not been evaluated from that point of view as yet. There are plans to do this.

HEGGENESS: One of the news reports of Gemini IV said that it was necessary to change the planned sleep-wakefulness cycle, because both astronauts wanted to sleep at the same time, and both wanted to go to sleep at their usual time of retiring.

BROWN: The subjective observations were that they were both in phase, but there are all sorts of reasons why this could have been, independent of any circadian rhythm.

BROBECK: Sometimes we forget how these rhythms interact. For example, if you put a dozen female animals in activity cages in a room where they are alone, eventually the twelve animals will come into the same cycle. They entrain one another by their activity, and, I guess, odor and other stimuli.

Maybe some of you have even seen this happen in infants. A mother eventually entrains her baby, because she does not like to get up every two or three hours to feed the baby, and so she establishes her rhythm in the baby. This is an unnatural situation, but it occurs all the time.

K. SCHWARZ: But are there not some inherent differences? If you look at any random population, there are people who start off very strongly in the morning, they are early risers and do their best work in the early part of the day; and there are other people who do not really get started until two o'clock in the afternoon. Then, there are night owls. These different behavioral cycles may be the result of early conditioning, more immediate psychological stimuli or some distinctive physiological pattern—but there can be no doubt these differences exist.

BROBECK: The length of the cycle is the same, isn't it?

K. SCHWARZ: Well, I think there are people who apparently need a lot more sleep than others.

BROBECK: It is conceivable that if these people were put in caves independently, they would be shown to have cycles of different length inherently, but as far as I know, there are not enough good data about this.

Ogden Nash's observation is the most pertinent, I think. He said that one kind marries the other.

K. SCHWARZ: You cannot shift circadian cycles around, at least not that part of the cyclic pattern which is inherent in an individual. It is my experience, for instance, that a "night" person cannot adapt at all to a typical "early morning-day" cycle. I have seen people who were married to each other and who tried very hard to adapt their cycles to each other, to no avail.

POLLARD: Have there not been some rather prolonged experiments with men kept in confinement on specified diets?

BROBECK: To follow their cycles?

POLLARD: Yes.

BROBECK: I do not know that anyone has purposely taken the man who wakes up slowly and the man who wakes up quickly and compared their free-running cycles. There are studies of the kind you have mentioned where you could get some idea of the variability of cycles of the population that was studied, but I do not believe they have had this particular purpose. I would guess from studies of laboratory animals and from what we see around us that if you have more than one subject, they are very likely going to entrain one another's cycles, but perhaps not on a twenty-four hour cycle. It might be a little off one way or the other, depending on unknown factors.

BROBECK: So there may be an identifiable rhythm that has a shorter period than the ordinary three-meal rhythm.

LIVINGSTON: Dr. Brobeck, you may be interested in the Sea Lab experiments that have just been completed off La Jolla, California.* The men tended to be very restless at night; they got up every two or three hours and raided the icebox. This was also their favorite occupation during the day.

They took in, by crude estimate, something like 3000 or 4000 calories per day and must have had a considerable expenditure of energy. Most aquanauts lost a little weight. They complained of broken sleep and unbroken appetite.

BARNES: Were they kept in a cool environment?

LIVINGSTON: They were too hot and too moist all of the time.

BARNES: How much of the time were they in the water?

LIVINGSTON: They were one or two hours a day in the water, I believe. They felt cold in the water.

K. SCHWARZ: I would like to come back to one primary point: the question of how circadian mechanisms are established. Our 24-hour daily rhythm is strictly conditioned—it is by habit, but it is normally adjusted to day and night; that is, to sunlight and no sunlight. That stimulus for the establishment and for the maintenance of the rhythm would not be there in space.

BROBECK: The entraining—that is, holding it at almost exactly 24 hours—depends upon the diurnal cycle in light and dark, but studies of men isolated in caves show that this rhythm persists in most subjects at something near 24 hours for a very surprising length of time.

K. SCHWARZ: In the Arctic and the Antarctic?

BROBECK: Yes, for months. There are a few instances of people who have lost their 24-hour cycle while they were in the cave, but these seem to be the odd ones. The usual response is that these things persist. The diurnal cycles that are built into lower animals are almost inextinguishable.

FREMONT-SMITH: What happened to those who lost their rhythms? Did they cease to eat for days at a time?

BROBECK: They took up new cycles of another length.

FREMONT-SMITH: They just changed the length of the cycle? They did not lose it?

---

* The Sea Lab experiments refer to Sea Lab II conducted under the aegis of the U. S. Navy from the surface ship Berkone under the direction of Dr. George Bond. The study, supported by the ONR (Office of Naval Research) and perhaps other parts of the Navy, was designed to test man's ability to live and work two hundred feet under the sea for extended periods of time.

BROBECK: It is a little hard to say whether it is diurnal rhythm or not when it becomes an 18-hour cycle.

MUNRO: This would emphasize the importance of knowing your man before you send him up, what he is likely to do.

FENN: Some of the cycles are much more persistent than others—I do not mean in different people, but in the same person. I talked about this both at New London, in the Naval Laboratory, and also at Hampstead, England, in the National Medical Research Institute—Dr. Edholm's laboratory. Both told me that, for example, the potassium cycle was very persistent compared to the body temperature cycles. Usually you excrete potassium in the daytime, and it diminishes at night. There is a regular cycle of potassium excretion and kidney function in general, but this cycle of excretion of potassium persists even though the night and day cycle changes. You deliberately enclose a man and control his night and day, or have him in a place where it is always night or always day, so that there is no guidance any more—

FREMONT-SMITH: Did you change his sleep cycle, and not change the potassium?

FENN: Yes. That is, the potassium cycle will lag behind, compared with other criteria. Some persist more than others do, and others will follow the light and dark very promptly.

POLLARD: How do men maintain circadian cycles on long submerged trips in submarines? Is this by association with others and the habits of eating?

REYNOLDS: I do not know of any relevant studies of people in submarines. There have been studies of people in submarines just off the dock in New London, submerged in a few feet of water, and it may be that the data are there, but I do not remember any analysis of it from the point of view of circadian rhythms.

There is work now under way by Aschoff of the Max Planck Institute. He has built some underground bunkers, and is doing very careful studies of circadian rhythms in humans. It is a job to maintain a really noncycle stimulus-free environment—if any of the operations in connection with care of the subjects follow a 24-hour cycle, or any recognizable submultiple of it, the subjects will cue onto that. It requires a very careful manipulation of the way you are handling the subjects, and they do have to be strictly isolated from other people, or entraining will persist.

ARNOLDI: Can I bring up an engineering viewpoint here? What you have been discussing pertains more specifically to a small free-running social group of a small number of people—one, two, or three—and ignores certain of the operational aspects of the space flight. In the case of any complex piece of mechanism, whether it is a submarine, a battleship—let us say, a squadron of jet airplanes, or a space vehicle which has a crew of more than three—perhaps five or ten—there will be operational requirements. There will be the need to maintain a regular series of watches. There will be need for coordination, for performance of duties which are arbitrarily set forth as a result of the well-defined mission involved, which will enforce some sort of an arbitrary schedule which might be the normal diurnal schedule on earth, or any other cycle.

Nevertheless, there will have to be such a cycle established as a matter of efficient utilization of a complex piece of equipment, completely aside from the convenience of the personnel's metabolism or other factors.

BROBECK: This is a problem that has been solved by the Navy in the submarines. I know about it only by hearsay, but I'm sure that you can get this information. The original complaint was that the men who were off duty were not able to sleep because they were disturbed by the men who were in the waking part of their cycle.

BROWN: That is true in space.

REYNOLDS: The source of the difficulty was that the Navy had adopted a system of "dogging the watch." It seemed that watches at particular hours of the day were preferable to other watches; and, in order that everybody have a fair shake, watches were shifted through the 24-hour period. This was a way of assuring that everybody was at the average minimum of alertness during a watch and was at an average minimum of sleepiness during a sleeping period. In other words, it could not have been arranged more unfortunately for gearing people to circadian cycles.

The Navy did this for something like 25 years. Finally, they were convinced that this was not a good thing, and switched over to a system that kept people on a more regular schedule, and it has been a lot better system.

BROBECK: You and I are expressing the same conclusion. I was going to say that what they did was to set up a condition where three different groups of men can run on three different schedules.

REYNOLDS: That's right.

ARNOLDI: Like three shifts in a factory.

BROBECK: It is even better than this because, you see, there is not the entraining of light and darkness that there is in the factory. In these nuclear submarines one man says it is day, and the other guy says it is night, or someplace in between. They just operate eating and feeding and work and sleep and recreation, each as if this were the normal diurnal cycle. Meanwhile the two other groups are going along on two other cycles separately.

ARNOLDI: Nevertheless, somebody—the submarine commander or in the GHQ someplace—does establish a 24-hour pattern. As far as I know, there has never been consideration of a 25-hour day on submarines, or something like that. These considerations have overridden biological characteristics, which might vary.

BROBECK: The human cycle is so easily entrained that I do not think this is going to be any problem, provided regularity exists. Even shift workers who have to change shifts have trouble working in factories. Many persons have this kind of difficulty; and they lose weight and get indigestion, and some of them get ulcers in the time that they are on a given shift. They just can not wait to be put over to another one. But if *everything* in their environment and schedule can be controlled, they will easily take up a new rhythm. I do not believe that this is really a problem in space flight.

REYNOLDS: Well, except that we do not know what may result from separation from the physical properties of the earth, if these stimulate circadian rhythms. There has been a fairly strong recommendation to NASA that we go beyond the influence of the earth, a distance of six or more radii away, and do studies of this nature completely removed from terrestrial influence.

There are not any firm plans to do this at the moment. There are some experiments proposed for the biosatellite.

Dehydration and Food Consumption

EPSTEIN: One point which has not been raised is the very close relation between hydration and hunger, and I think it should be emphasized. I am confident that we can rely on healthy young men to maintain themselves in good nutritional balance if they are offered a reasonably wide range of foods, none of which is frankly unpalatable.

One thing that may interfere is dehydration, which is a very potent anorexigenic agent. It decreases hunger very rapidly and very severely, and produces an obvious positive feedback; that is, the thirsty man does not eat. He, therefore, does not drink. He becomes thirstier, and he does not eat.

FREMONT-SMITH: You mean, the thirsty man avoids drink?

EPSTEIN: No, if the animal, or man, is thirsty, he will eat less. Eating itself is a great stimulus to drinking, and if he has eaten less, he may also consequently drink less and become more dehydrated.

FREMONT-SMITH: Even if water is available to him?

EPSTEIN: If he is not drinking the water, which was, as I understand it, a problem in these short-term Mercury flights—one simple way that hydration can be assured is by offering very dilute foods, sort of watery milkshakes, watery Metrecal—very palatable. You can either think of it as a dilute food or as a palatable liquid.

FREMONT-SMITH: A very nauseating dilute food or a very palatable liquid, depending on how you think about it.

EPSTEIN: Well, I do not think it is nauseating. I prefer them, but, I mean, again if we knew the food preferences of the astronaut before he was out of our control, and if there were some means of making available to him foods he enjoyed, I believe he would be well hydrated, and this would avoid what I consider to be the most likely cause of a failure in his nutrition —that is, dehydration.

Taste and Odor

FENN: How about your animals that are deprived of sensations of smell and taste. Do they select the foods that they are accustomed to, or will they select the things they need? What do they tell us about this problem?

EPSTEIN: Nothing that I can see, I am sorry to say. My experiments,[89] tell me that the rat is an excellent regulator of nutrients in the absence of taste and smell—that is, in the absence of the flavor of the food he is eating. They do not tell us anything about selection, because in order to study selection you have to force the animals to make choices. They have a single bar that they manipulate in order to maintain a single food. It is a Greenstein diet [composed of highly purified ingredients].

It is in the area of selection, and of incentive to eat and motivation to work for food, that the oropharyngeal sensations are important, and not in the phenomenon of regulation—that is, the metering of intake to meet a nutritional need.

BROBECK: It is important in determining what he will eat, but not how much he will eat of it.

EPSTEIN: Exactly.

Choice of Test Animals

POLLARD: Are rats the best experimental animal with which to study such matters as eating habits?

EPSTEIN: I do not think the rat is the ideal animal for all psychological testing, particularly when you are asking essentially human questions, like problem solution and levels of intelligence, and so on, but when it comes to the regulation of food intake and food selection and the study of meals—and rats have meals—and the relationships between food and water intake, the rat is the animal of choice.

POLLARD: Have you tried others?

BROBECK: The rat is a precision machine for this purpose.

BROWN: Do you say this because of the reproducibility of the data, or because he is so similar to man in some respects?

EPSTEIN: Both. He is a regular beast and a particular beast, and he is like us in all of the important phenomena, except in his nocturnal habit.

K. SCHWARZ: There is one physiological aspect in which the rat is very different, and that is in its biological time equivalence. If we fast a rat overnight, let us say for 18 hours, the result is not at all equivalent to that of an overnight fast in the human. A day's fast in the rat amounts to 10 to 17 days of fasting in man, at least with respect to many of the variables which deserve consideration.

EPSTEIN: An overnight fast for a shrew can be fatal.

Food Storage versus Food Generation

SCHWEIGERT: I would like to speak to a question that seems to come up right along relative to this closed system thing. It is implied that we could not take conventional foods and water for the couple of years that are envisioned in future space ship missions, so that appetite regulation is going to have to be evaluated in terms of unconventional foods, I deduce. Is that an incorrect deduction?

BROBECK: I think this may be true, and if it is, then I recommend that it be done before the man is sent off into space.

I wish we knew a lot more about the fundamental science, but if we have to get along without it and solve the problems in a purely practical way I think it should be done before the man is put into the space capsule.

REYNOLDS: After the session yesterday, we had a discussion of the amount of weight that would be involved, in pounds per man per day of dehydrated foods. It turned out that food weight would be in the order of seven tons for a thousand-day trip for ten men,* which struck me as a remarkably low quantity of solid material. That is less than the weight of oxygen which you would have to carry.

Frankly, it gave me a little different perspective on this.

SCHWEIGERT: I do not have any idea of payloads, but it seems to me it is not unreasonable. It is?

REYNOLDS: I do not think it is.

BROBECK: It is not unreasonable to send up [a three-year supply of] dehydrated conventional foods?

REYNOLDS: Offhand, it sounds like a lot smaller weight penalty than I would have thought was involved.

BROBECK: This is after you get the water out of it. About two thirds or three fourths of the weight of most foods is water.

REYNOLDS: You are going to have to recycle the water anway.

K. SCHWARZ: Figures such as we are discussing are presented in the report on the Conference on Nutrition in Space and Related Waste Problems.[1] Utilizing conventional storage, they calculate the weight requirement for ten men for one year to be 70000 to 90000 lbs., and the volume is given

* Weight of dehydrated foods to yield 2800 kcal. is about 600 g., if fat provides about 35 to 40% of the calories and allowance is made for residual water, minerals and nondigestible constituents. Weight of packaging material is not included. Ed.

as approximately 1800 cubic feet [for the entire life support system: food, oxygen and water].

SCHWEIGERT: Then would somebody explain why the necessity of this closed system for providing his food is being talked about so much?

KRAUSS: I think I could at least come close to answering that.

In a closed system we are concerned with provision for gas exchange as well as food consumption. We are thinking of utilizing microorganisms for the production of oxygen and removal of CO_2. The by-product of such a system is fat, carbohydrate, protein, and vitamins in the cells of the organism which must grow in order to effect the gas exchange.

That organism, theoretically at least, may be part of the food supply, if not all of the food supply. The process of getting adequate gas exchange means that you have to produce an organism, and then the question is: what do you do with the organism?

The logical thing is to eat it. You might as well use the by-product because you have it.

Could I ask a question with regard to this matter of acceptability? I assume that the discussion so far indicates that you could come up with a balanced diet, a bland diet of some sort that could be fed to the astronaut. Such a diet, similar to a can of Metrecal, but balanced—not a reducing diet—could be fed to him three times a day indefinitely. However I believe that you are saying this could seriously affect his efficiency and would have some psychological reaction which is very bad for him. Could not one assume that you might come up with just one standard formula that is quite acceptable to him and keep him on that indefinitely?

BROBECK: This is conceivable, but we simply do not have the data. This is the kind of experiment that I think ought to be done.

BARNES: Dr. E. H. Ahrens* and his associates at the Rockefeller University in New York, have kept patients for over a year exclusively on a formula type diet.

KRAUSS: So there is really no fundamental objection to this, other than a slight psychological one?

MAYER: And what is more, it would appear, from animal work, that the longer you go on and the greater the food deprivation, the greater is the certainty that, as long as the diet is not too objectionable, human beings will regulate their body weight on this diet.

K. SCHWARZ: They may even come to like it. They may be conditioned to it.

BROBECK: Dr. Mayer and I are going to differ a little bit here. It is true that when an individual is deprived of food, he becomes less discriminating

* Personal communication.

about what he eats; but so far as I know it is not true that when a man is deprived of other kinds of sensory stimuli that he will become less discriminating about food. I think that all the evidence is that he will become more discriminating (FIGURE 5).

MAYER: We must remember that all of us have been on a formula diet for many months of our lives, when we started out, and many children are in effect on a formula diet for a year, at a time when food is the major stimulus.

FREMONT-SMITH: It is not the major stimulus, because they die if they do not get the emotional stimulus. What usually is associated is that feeding and loving go together for the infant.

I think this is a very important distinction to make.

BROBECK: I do not mean to discount the formula diet. You will find in the paper I wrote for the Hardy monograph [70] that I recommended the use of these simple diets extensively.

Ask me "what's for dinner"
just once more and I'm
gonna let yuh have it!

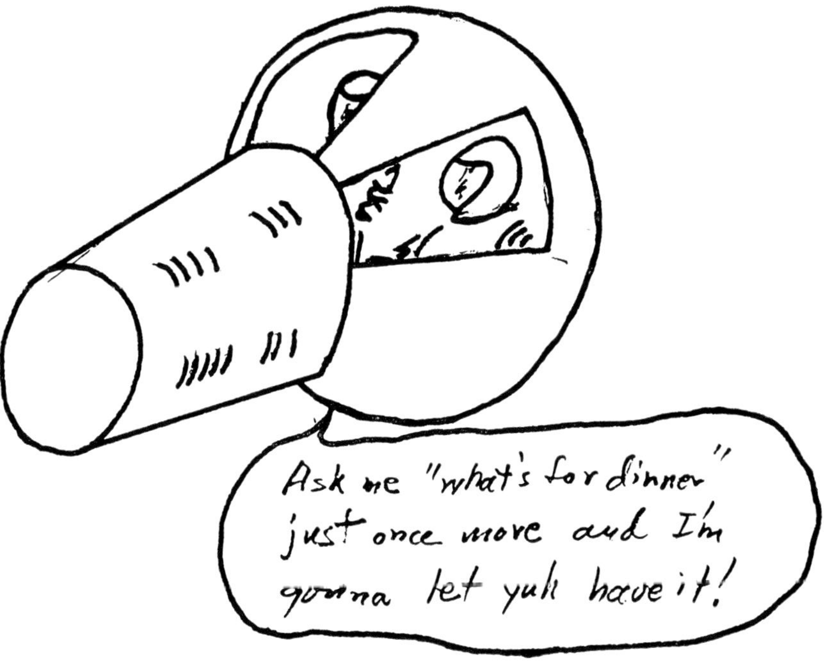

FIGURE 5. Walter Arnoldi's evaluation of food attitudes in space flight.

D. SCHWARZ: I think there is another factor here, and that is the waste disposal. There is a big difference in waste disposal between a conventional diet and a reasonably good formula diet.

SCHWEIGERT: Well, that is a refinement of even a conventional food, in contrast to a closed system.

K. SCHWARZ: Well, what is a conventional food? You can take it and refine it partway, or further and further until you have minimized your waste disposal problem, which is considered to be a fairly serious problem for long missions.

MAYER: From what Dr. Gustafsson and Dr. Mossel are going to tell us this afternoon, flora may become very different, depending on the ration. This may be a strong argument for beginning to feed people their space ration quite a bit before they go on their space trip.

BROBECK: I think you could suggest that if an astronaut wishes to be in a two-year program, one of the conditions of the program should be that he eats during the training what he is going to get in the capsule.

V. INTESTINAL MICROFLORA AND GERMFREE LIFE

Discussion Leader:

BENGT E. GUSTAFSSON
Department of Germfree Research
Karolinska Institutet
Stockholm, Sweden

GUSTAFSSON: May I begin by saying how happy I am to be here.

I believe the two most hazardous things that the astronaut brings into his capsule on an extended flight over several months or years are his brain and his intestinal flora. I will discuss some problems concerning the microbial aspects today.

I will first talk about endosymbiosis. Then I think we should discuss the intestinal flora in monogastric animals, how well it is defined and not defined, and how it might be influenced by the diet and other factors. We will briefly consider the germfree technique and review the characteristics of germfree animals. I will also try to emphasize that these charactertics might be found in the ordinary, conventional animal with a so-called normal intestinal flora. Finally we will talk about which minimal flora is necessary to compensate for eventually developing germfree characteristics and deficiency symptoms. The big question here, of course, is if such germfree characteristics or deficiency symptoms could occur in man in space, if the intestinal flora for one reason or another is changing or "drifting" in the astronaut.

All of us are in contact with and harboring enormous numbers of bacteria. It has been calculated that only one out of a thousand of bacterial strains is what is generally termed pathogenic.

The role played by this abundant microbial flora has been the focus of many investigations since the time of Pasteur, and he postulated that life without bacteria would not be possible. The first studies along these lines were really started during the last ten years of the last century.

Symbiosis

There is a lot of evidence collected, however, on the relationship between the so-called nonpathogenes or saprophytes in other fields of research.

The entomologists have for a long time studied the cooperation between bacteria and insects, and they have used this term "endosymbiosis" as a label for the interaction between microbiota and the host organism.

As a matter of introduction here I will show you some figures about endosymbiosis in insects. Histological examination of insects will reveal that some organs always contain pure strains of bacteria. These cells are usually closely related to the intestinal tract, and techniques have been worked out to make these animals sterile—germfree—very easily, by heating the eggs, for example. If you do that, the larva (*a*) in FIGURE 6 does not grow. The larva (*b*) is also germfree, of the same age, and has the same nutrient medium as (*a*) but the B vitamins have been added as yeast extracts to the medium. Now the germfree larva shows almost the same normal growth as the nonsterile larva (*c*) of the bread bug, *Sitodrepa panicea*.

In all these insects with endosymbiosis there are special organs, mycetomes, with large vacuolated cells containing the symbiotic microorganisms.

The bacteria are intracellular with a high degree of adaptation to the host tissue. This makes them very difficult to cultivate under ordinary laboratory conditions.

The host is in most cases of endosymbiosis entirely dependent on the symbiotic microorganism, and very intricate mechanisms ensure that the symbion is propagated from one host generation to the other. In many cases the ovum is the carrier. In FIGURE 7 there is an other example. The female *Coptosoma* is putting a pure culture from its intestinal flora close to the newly laid egg. The first action of the newly hatched larva is to

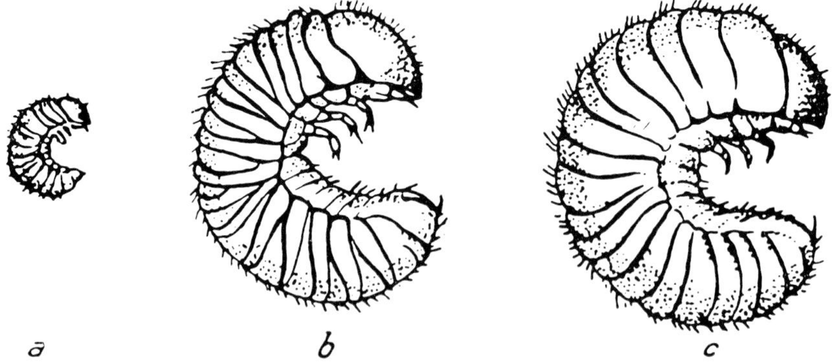

FIGURE 6. Effect of symbiont removal in *Sitodrepa panicea L.* (a) Ten-week-old larva without symbionts kept sterile on pea-meal; (b) larva of the same age without symbionts kept sterile in pea-meal and dried yeast; (c) symbiont-containing larva of the same age as control. From: Buchner, P., Endosymbiosis of animals with plant microorganisms, Interscience Publishers, 1965.

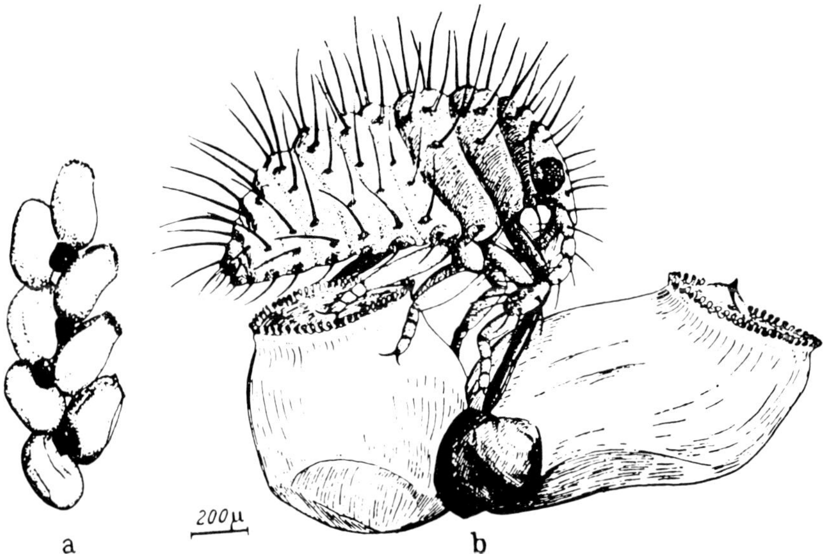

FIGURE 7. *Coptosoma scutellatum Geoffr.* (a) Eggs with bacteria-filled cocoons added by the female. (b) A newly hatched larva sucking the contents from the symbiont-containing capsule. From: Koch, A. in Medizinische Grundlagenforschung, G. Thieme, 1962.

suck these organisms. If this is prohibited, the larva will die from the lack of symbiosis with the microorganism in question.

The herbivores are another good example of endosymbiosis with the very complex interrelationship in the rumen—with constant symbiosis between different members of a large population of microorganisms and, in turn, with those and the host.

Human Intestinal Flora

When man is considered, one must keep in mind that intestinal bacteria are present not only in the colon and the cecum but also in the lower part of the ileum and—not to forget—in the mouth. The number of bacteria in these parts of the body is very large. It is up to 10^{10} bacteria per gram content, or even higher sometimes. You will also recall that at least half of the fecal matter consists of dead or living bacteria.

In the mouth there is so much bacteria found that it has been calculated that each of us swallows 1.0 g. of bacterial matter per day, which is produced in the mouth. The mouth flora has been overlooked in the discussion of microbial synthesis of accessory food factors. The fat-soluble vitamin K, produced by the mouth flora, is of much greater importance to the host than that produced in the large intestine, as it is easily absorbed due to the action of the bile.

FREMONT-SMITH: Is there a relationship between the bacteria in the mouth and those in the intestine?

GUSTAFSSON: Yes, very much.

FREMONT-SMITH: It looks as if you had the rest of the intestine sterile, but it is not sterile, is it?

GUSTAFSSON: Well, there is debate on that. It depends on the method you are using. There are bacteria all the way up.

They are obligate anaerobes and sometimes very hard to subculture. They are mentioned very briefly in Bergey's Manual, which is the most comprehensive handbook for the classification of bacteria. The intestinal flora also contains large numbers of *Lactobacilli,* which are very badly classified and defined. If you ask a medical man what is present in the intestinal tract, he will say *E. coli,* and he finds *E. coli* down here, but you will hear from Dr. Mossel pretty soon that he is wrong.

In FIGURE 8 I have tried to demonstrate that most of the intestinal flora

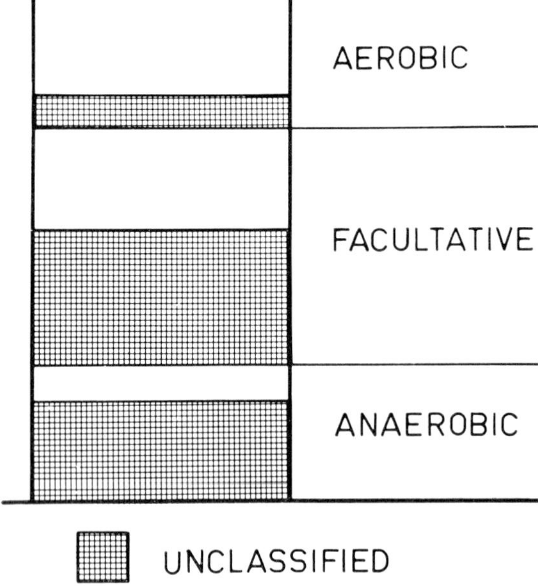

FIGURE 8. Most strains of the bacteria in the intestinal contents are unclassified and belong to the facultative or anaerobic groups.

consists of unclassified material and that many of the strains are anaerobic. This means that the methods used in the collection of fecal samples and the following analysis have to be carefully observed. I now think I will leave the floor to Dr. Mossel, who is an expert in these matters.

MOSSEL: Well, on this occasion of my first appearance in the floor show, may I also express how much I appreciate being here and having an opportunity to tell you what we have found these last years about the intestinal flora of adult man and the possible implications for submarine navigation and space flying.

The things that I am going to tell you are the fruit of long research, carried out not only by my group, but also by the Departments of Pediatrics and Biochemistry under my colleagues Weijers and van de Kamer; in fact the material I will present is barely one third my own work.

In TABLE 9, we have very roughly brought together what is known about the viable intestinal flora of healthy children and adults. I do not know anything about pigs and rats and mice. These figures are, let me say, the median ranges for these various groups of organisms which one may encounter in the intestinal contents.

What we examine is stools—freshly voided stools, immediately brought under strictly anaerobic conditions, because, as Dr. Gustafsson said, this is very essential. Most of our intestinal organisms need a low oxygen partial pressure in order to survive; many of the older workers fell into this pit, in that they analyzed stools which were too old and therefore too much oxygenated to give the poor obligately anaerobic organisms a chance to survive.

FREMONT-SMITH: Must you have it immediately anaerobic?

TABLE 9

VIABLE INTESTINAL FLORA OF HEALTHY CHILDREN AND ADULTS [90]

	Species or type	Count per g. wet faeces
Saccharolytic flora	*Lactobacillus bifidus*	10^9 to 10^{10}
	Lactobacillus acidophilus	10^7 to 10^9
	Butyribacterium rettgeri	cne*
	Veillonella alcalescens	cne
Saccharoproteolytic flora	Bacteroides	10^{10} to 10^{11}
	Enterobacteriaceae	10^6 to 10^8
	Lancefield D streptococci	10^4 to 10^7
	Clostridia	10^3 to 10^6
	Staphylococcus aureus	10^1 to 10^3

* Count not yet exactly established

MOSSEL: Immediately. So the moment after it is voided—and this is a lot of work for the nurses in the Pediatric Section, as you can imagine—it is diluted 1:10 with a prechilled, anaerobic protective diluent, refrigerated to +2°C, and then examined bacteriologically. Unless we preserve the stool in this anaerobic state, we might lose a considerable and essential part of the organisms.

We brought together in this little Table (9) the things we know for sure and so we had often to indicate cne—count not yet exactly, or not yet at all, established.

You see, even the organisms which we know rather well we cannot always enumerate; so it becomes, I hope, explicit from this Table how elementary our knowledge in this field is.

FIGURE 9 brings the same data, but now in a histogram version. As you may see from the title of this figure, we have rebaptized the normal, healthy ecological conditions in the ileocecal region of healthy people as *eubacteriosis*. It is as good as any other word, I think. When something significant happens in this region we talk about a disturbed intestinal ecology or *dysbacteriosis*.

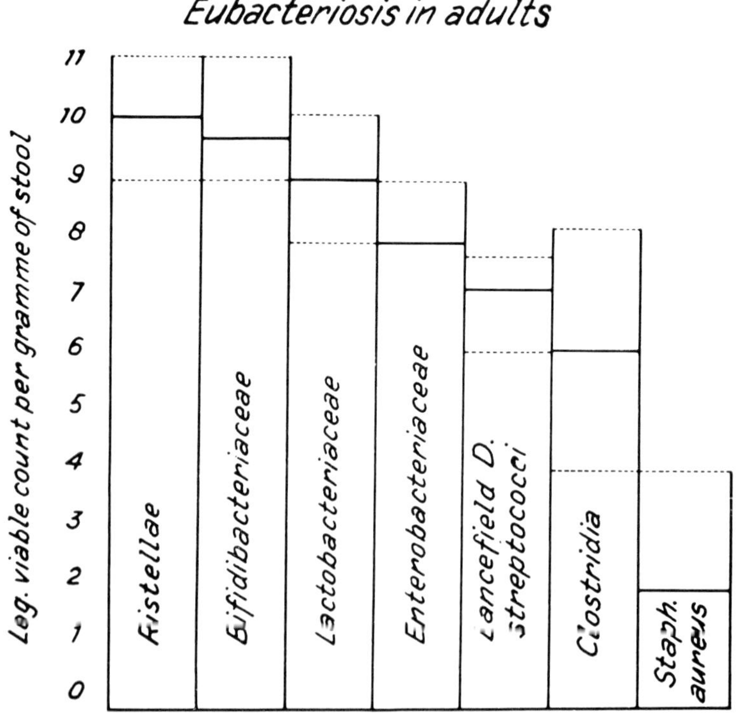

FIGURE 9. Eubacteriosis in adults.[90]

What we did here is the normal thing in clinical sciences, giving the median values for the number of organisms per one gram of stool as we know they are at present, along with the variation seen under physiological conditions. Some numbers are extremely high. Organisms often indicated as *Ristellae,* which is the modern word for the faecal types among the bacteria grouped as *Bacteroides,* are in the region of log viable count per gram of stool somewhere around nine to eleven. When you compare these figures with those for our poor *E. coli,* of which log viable count is only $10^8 - 10^9$, their abundance may be one thousandth of the most numerous enteric organisms. So, how wrong is our average clinical colleague who says the predominant organism in the stool of healthy man is *E. coli* or *Proteus!*

Next, there are the other things that Dr. Gustafsson has already mentioned. Note that *Staphyloccus aureus* has a very minor position in all normal stools; however, the symptom of danger is there as soon as *Staph. aureus* goes up. We know that this may often be fatal, because it might produce an enterocolitis which may take the patient's life.

As a matter of fact, we are not primarily interested in the numbers and types of organisms though, but rather in their metabolic patterns. What do they do, and why?

Tables 10 and 11 present the most recent elementary summary of the biochemical activities of the enteric bacteria of primary significance.

Fremont-Smith: Where was this published?

Mossel: In part in *Nutrition Abstracts and Reviews 35:* 591 (1965),[90] but new findings have become available since and these have been incorporated in the two Tables.

Our approach, however, was very elementary. We just tried to find parameters for saccharolytic activity and proteolytic activity; the latter, as far as we are informed—gelatinase and tryptophanase activity.

This is roughly what we know at present. As you see, often the genera or species cannot be exactly specified because we just do not know what is going on.

For instance, the enteric organism *Veillonella alcalescens,* is wonderful to put in an academic review, but one can hardly isolate it from human stools by modern bacteriological techniques. It is listed because we know that, together with *Bacteroides* spp., it may form propionic acid, which we detected in considerable quantities in stools—but for the rest we have not got the slightest idea about the importance of *Veillonella* in eubacteriosis. It may also well be that part of the propionic acid found in stools, stems from methane-producing, obligately anaerobic bacteria.

All this originates from our ideas, arrived at, about five years ago, that this approach of purely bacteriological techniques—counts and dif-

TABLE 10

GENERAL METABOLIC ACTIVITY OF INTESTINAL BACTERIA [90]

Species or type	Saccharolytic activity Acids produced					Gelatinase and tryptophanase activity
	Lactic	Formic	Acetic	Other	$CO_2 + H_2$	
Lactobacillus acidophilus	++	—	+	—	—	—
Lactobacillus bifidus	++	—	+	—	—	—
Lancefield D streptococci	++	+	+	—	—	d *
Enterobacteriaceae	+	+	+	—	d	d
Bacteroides	+	d	+	propionic * butyric *	±	d
Clostridia	+	+	++	butyric	++	+++
Staphylococcus aureus	++	—	—	—	—	+
Butyribacterium rettgeri	—	—	+	butyric caproic	—	—
Veillonella alcalescens	—	—	+	propionic	+	—

* Different reactions shown by different genera or species

TABLE 11

NUMERICAL DATA ON THE FORMATION OF VOLATILE ALIPHATIC ACIDS BY INTESTINAL BACTERIA [90]

Group of organisms	Number of strains studied	Median values (%) of volatile acids			
		Formic	Acetic	Propionic	Butyric
Ristellae	42	5	67	28	—
R. convexa	1	—	50	11	39
R. putredinis	1	4	30	13	30
Bif. bifidum	10	2	98	—	—
Cl. perfringens	13	2	72	—	26
Cl. sporogenes	4	—	34	—	53
Veill. alcalescens	3	—	40	60	—

ferentiation—would not get us very far. FIGURE 10 may help you to understand why.

Pathogenicity of Enteric Organisms

We know from pathology that the gastrointestinal region and the occurrences we are really interested in, are in the ileocecal area. That is where the nonabsorbed nutrients out of our diet and the intestinal bacteria get together and either make us sick or keep us healthy, as far as enteric diseases are concerned.

Perhaps this is the proper moment to say that we will not discuss any classical infectious disease like *Salmonellosis* or *Shigellosis,* where an aggressive, invasive organism may disturb the whole pattern. We are just interested, for space flight and for submarine naval prolems, in people who are kept under normal, noninfectious conditions. I mean, it is just the classical procedure in preventive medicine to keep these factors out. Is that not so?

GUSTAFSSON: Some of the *Clostridia* that we find in clinically healthy individuals could be pathogenic.

MOSSEL: They are potential pathogens, I agree immediately; but I wanted to climinate from the discussion the classical pathogens like *Salmonella, Shigella,* hepatitis virus, and so forth.

GUSTAFSSON: I just wanted to get on the record that even if you get a healthy astronaut into the capsule, and he then would get a wound, for example, this might be infected by pathogens from his intestinal tract. Such a condition could be very difficult to handle under the circumstances.

MOSSEL: How right you are!

POLLARD: Is there any such thing as a nonpathogenic agent?

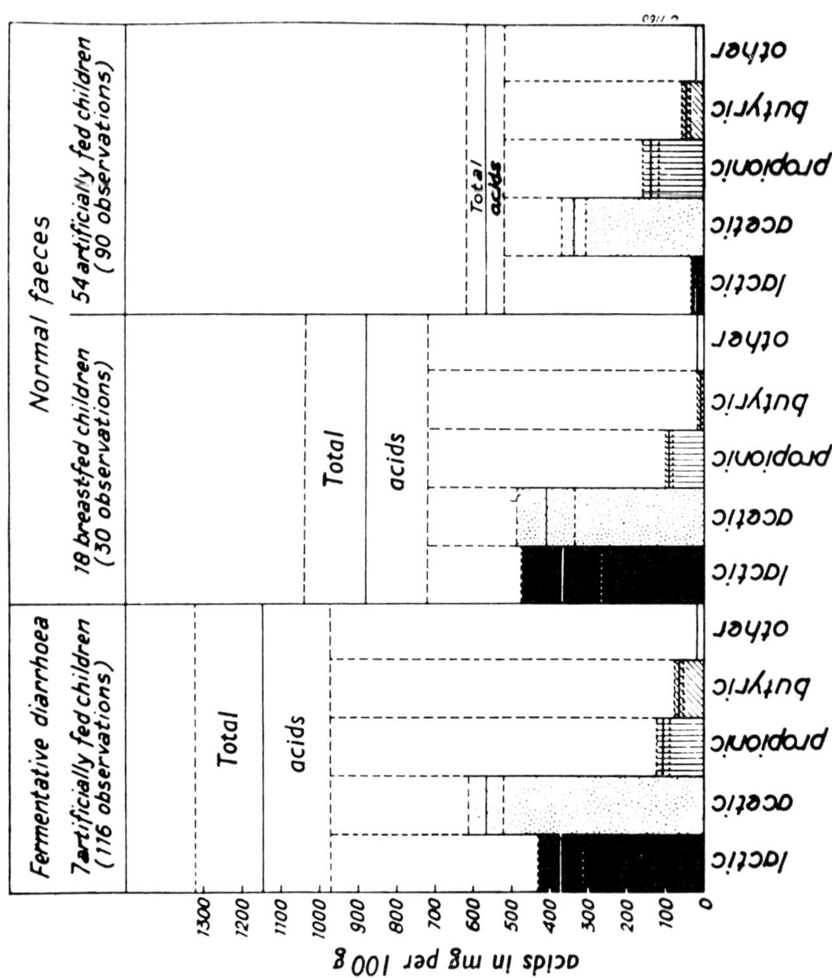

FIGURE 10. Comparative figures on acids in feces of breastfed and artificially fed children.[8]

MOSSEL: Under the conditions which we are considering here, I do think so, yes.

POLLARD: I am saying this with a purpose in mind, because it depends on the resistance of the host. The most benign agent can become pathogenic if the host resistance drops.

GUSTAFSSON: Or if the soil becomes so favorable for one bacteria that it outgrows the others.

POLLARD: I think all organisms are potentially pathogenic.

FREMONT-SMITH: Facultatively pathogenic.

MOSSEL: If so defined, this is agreed.

MUNRO: Quite a lot of people carry *Staph. aureus* in the nose. Do the organisms found in the feces come from the nasal bacteria, which are able to reach the bottom of the tract, or do they in fact multiply within the—

MOSSEL: All healthy adults and children indeed harbor *Staph. aureus* in their stools, but the significance of this depends on what numbers per gram of stool. You may have one in 100 gram, one in 10 gram, or one in a gram, which are very low figures. What is decisive here, is, in effect, the old "seed and soil" idea of Pasteur. As long as microbes are somewhere and they do not find a soil too favorable to proliferate—and I am now referring to *Staph. aureus* under intestinal anaerobic conditions—nothing will happen to the patient or to healthy individuals. But, may the Lord forefend that you ever get an outgrowth of this *Staph. aureus* in the intestinal environment—for instance, after antibiotic chemoprophylaxis before abdominal surgery. Then, most of the other organisms may have been eliminated, an almost pure culture of *Staph. aureus* may arise, with nothing to keep it under check, and this will result in what we call enterocolitis. This is a dreadful disease, because the enterotoxin formed by the pathogenic staphylococci will then be absorbed down in that colonic region, and this may kill the patient within 48 hours.

I said that we were interested, as a matter of fact, in what is happening microbiologically in the ileocecal region. This is what we are looking for. When we examine stools, however, we get data on (*1*) this material *after* having been exposed also to the colonic and anorectal areas, and, obviously many things may change then in this initial microflora; (*2*) numbers of organisms without exact data on their *activity,* which may be quite variable.

When trying to obtain the information of real clinical importance we remembered a word from the Gospel: "From the fruits they shall judge the tree."

As a matter of fact, the bacteria which have developed in the ileocecal area will have carried out certain biochemical reactions to a certain extent; the concentrations of the various products of these reactions (metabolites) are not likely to be changed essentially by passing through the colonic and rectal areas. Hence, if we examine stools properly in a chemical way, we might say: Look, here are quite some apples, hence somewhere there has been an actively blooming apple tree; whereas that looks like the harvest from a small pear tree.

And that is why we now make our *biochemical* approach to what is happening in the ileocecal region. I like particularly to give you a special example of what we think we have done. It refers to our studies of the eternal question, which has nothing to do with space research, of the differences between breast-fed and artificially fed children. We know that there are differences. Cultural methods gave us some clue, but not sufficiently so.

EPSTEIN: Can I interject a methodological question?

To get a more direct answer to the question of what is going on in the critical area of the ileocecum, why can you not employ all of the healthy appendices that are removed from humans in surgery?

MOSSEL: Because our professional gastroenterologists issue a warning that the so-called healthy appendices removed from so-called healthy people, do not at all represent a physiological state. There is first of all the indication: Why was the laparotomy done?

Secondly, there is the laparotomy itself, and we will later go into that. Such an intervention will certainly influence the pattern of secretions which might, in turn, influence considerably what has happened in the ileocecal region.

EPSTEIN: I recall, for instance, on the Gynecological Service it is routine to remove the appendix when a woman is undergoing hysterectomy. This is not, I mean, a case in which you have gastrointestinal disease.

MOSSEL: No, but goodness! The material which one collects in the course of a hysterectomy is certainly not representing the physiological state. The presurgery treatments, the anesthetic supplies, and similar things might seriously interfere with the secretory patterns, therefore modify the soil, and by that token modify the performance of the enteric seeds, do you not think so?

FREMONT-SMITH: In other words, there are complications within complications.

Still, it seems to me, it would give you—and I am sure you probably have done something—it would give you another approach which would be interesting to compare with what you get at the rectum.

MOSSEL: Right.

EPSTEIN: What about the use of healthy people dying, of traffic accidents—head injuries?

MOSSEL: There are some agonal changes in mortal accidents, which may affect the intestinal area, so that what we see post-mortem may be only an approximation of what is happening in a functioning, continuous culture, as the healthy ileocecal region is.

RAHN: But are you not also guessing by your method too?

MOSSEL: Well, we are still guessing, yes.

RAHN: So which guess is better, the direct approach, or—?

MOSSEL: We think our biochemical guess is better, because we do not interrupt a physiological cycle, and we just examine for metabolites.

Of course, these metabolites may be remetabolized—do you know what I mean? The initial metabolites may be metabolized in the course of being forwarded through the colon.

The results presented in FIGURE 10 are the ones referred to earlier, stemming from our pediatric research. You see, these are the stools of eighteen breast-fed children, and those of 54 artificially fed children. Our biochemist has determined all the volatile acids and lactic acid. The result was a wonderful difference. The breast-fed children had a lot of lactic and rather some acetic and propionic acid. The artificially fed children have almost no lactic acid, almost the same or slightly less acetic, have a significantly increased propionic acid, as well as butyric acid level, while the other metabolites are almost the same.

So, our clinical impression of the differences between breast-fed children and artificially fed children is reflected properly by a fully significant shift in the metabolites; this then gave us some confidence to carry on with our metabolic, rather than purely bacteriological, approach.

We have also studied what might be the bacteriology and the biochemistry of diarrhea in some adult cases. We have found that the following forces may in principle be operative (FIGURE 11). There may be challenging of the normal tolerance; for instance, someone is eating rather much of a certain carbohydrate. Now, for either physiological or pathological reasons, his absorption mechanism just cannot cope with all this carbohydrate. It escapes partly from absorption and therefore appears in the ileocecal region. Here it is fermented and produces a lot of lactic acid; this irritates the mucosa in this region, and a fermentative diarrhea may be the result.

GUSTAFSSON: Metchnikoff would not have liked that statement.

MOSSEL: Why not? Too much lactic acid may do harm, just as excesses generally do.

We have also seen cases where the secretion of mucus in the higher ileum, the region of absorption, prevented complete absorption of carbohydrate, or where there was a disturbance of the absorption of the same carbohydrate by the cell wall capillaries; there again we got supernormal

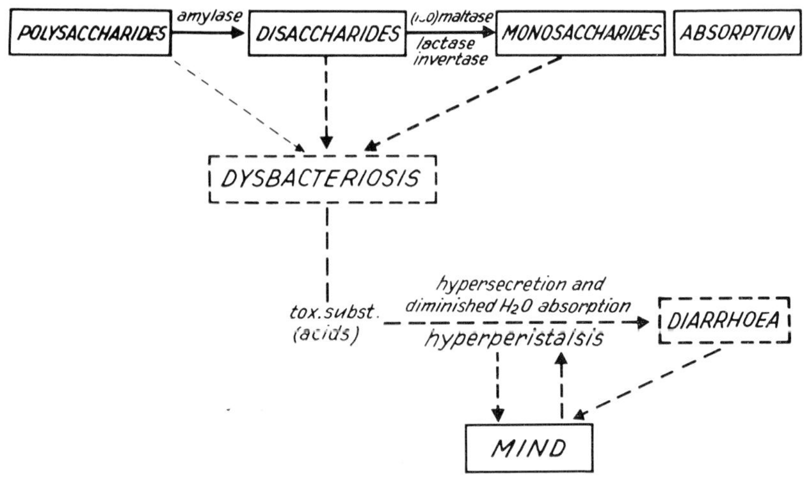

FIGURE 11. Fermentative diarrhea.[90]

concentrations of this carbohydrate in the ileocecal region, breakdown by microorganisms which immediately react to a change in their soil—you see, as the soil changes favorably, they go up in numbers; it is always the same—and we may get diarrhea.

I will leave out all of the pathology, but we had quite a few interesting cases. For instance one where a man, after [ileal] resection, got difficulties any time he was eating ice cream. We investigated the case and found that, due to this resection, the surface of the area of absorption had been reduced to such an extent that the patient could not cope any more with a normal amount of sucrose and lactose present in our Netherlandish ice cream, and so *he* got fermentative diarrhea, but other consumers did not.

Well, then we get into all those things which are determined by increased peristalsis, by inadequate phosphorylation due to drug administration, and so forth. To summarize, in fermentative diarrheas characterized by insufficient absorption of sugars, the soil is changed favorably for saccharolytic organisms. This flora will thereupon grow out and produce much lactic acid and in this way make the patient a diarrhoeic.

May I make it clear that these are, as Dr. Gustafsson said, the things which might occur in the space capsule *without* the introduction of any classical extrinsic pathogenic organisms. It is just the man's own microflora coming out of control.

Where putrefactive diarrhea occurs in the absence or presence of an invasive enteropathogen we have the impression the proteolysis may originate from the presence in the ileocecal region of either proteins or peptides, which normally do not occur in that region (FIGURE 12). This will, then, lead to a copious development of a proteolytic flora, which we have been able to identify to a certain extent. This flora then starts a vicious cycle. The first effect is that several products of proteolytic breakdown of peptides are going to irritate the enteric mucosa. This leads to more available amino acid and hence putrefaction and also to the phenomenon of resorption of metabolites such as the biogenic amines. This all results in a deterioration of the patient's general health, as we know it so well in those forms of proteolytic diarrhea.

Let me add a detail on these biogenic amines. It was noted some years ago that eating cheese could be causally associated with the onset of—occasionally lethal—attacks of acute hypertension, headaches, palpitation and flushing in patients suffering from depression and therefore treated with monoamineoxidase (MAO) inhibitors, such as iproniazed. The amine tyramine was eventually identified as the causative agent. Horwitz et al.[91] showed that as little as *ca.* 5 mg. of tyramine, corresponding with 20 g. of certain types of cheeses, may produce the type of attacks in MAO-inhibitor-treated patients just mentioned.

We think that a similar mechanism might be operative in patients suffering from prolonged putrefactive diarrhea. Due to the existence of the erosive lesions in the mucosa cells mentioned, these may produce less MAO. This, in turn, would lead to an unphysiological level of biogenic amines in the lower intestinal lumen while the simultaneously present increased absorption does the rest.

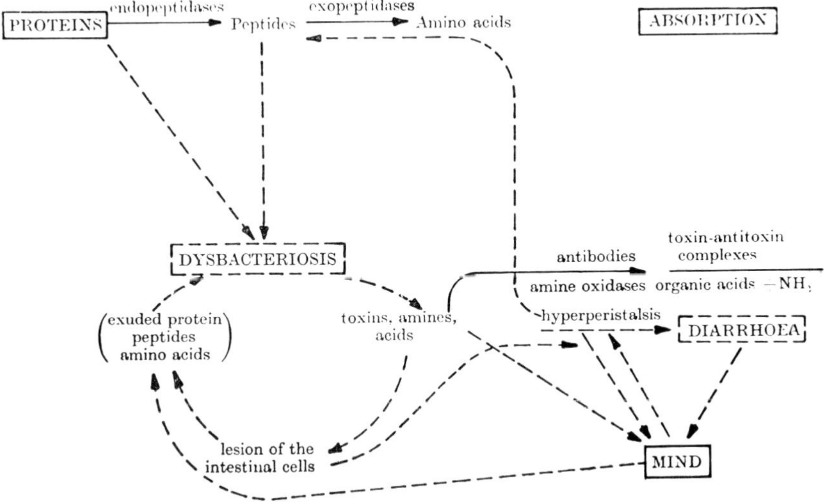

FIGURE 12. Putrefactive diarrhea.[90]

Hence, in case of fermentative dysbacteriosis we observe that people just have diarrhea; in addition they may have some pain in the perianal region, because those acids erode slightly, but they will not generally be sick, just pass more stools. However, people who have a proteolytic dysbacteriosis will normally have all types of complaints. If I may use the word, they feel lousy. They are not fit to go on duty. Now, how is a young medical officer going to establish that this man is sick? When he applies his little bit of routine examination of the stools of those patients, he will not find any pathogens; so next comes the verdict: This man is in good condition. However, we know now that he is sick. Even when we have made the patient fast, or if he takes only tea and toast (the classical treatment in the British Navy), the patient's proteolytic diarrhea may carry on automatically; because, once the lesions have occurred, the lumen-wall cells of the intestinal mucosa may take care of supplying enough protein, and keep the pathological process going.

GUSTAFSSON: What is the cause, in your mind, for the dysbacteriosis that you have been discussing?

MOSSEL: Either proteins or peptides may come primarily to the ileocecal region. It depends on the quantity and on the amino acid composition. If you have not got the precursors for those highly pharmacologically active amines, you will not have the most serious problem. A little bit of glycine only, for instance, would not do too much harm, provided only a limited amount of corrosive metabolites is formed.

GUSTAFSSON: There is a good range of security here, because, as has been shown by Borgström and his colleagues,[92] the proteins are absorbed in the first 75 cm. of the intestinal tract, and you have almost 2 m. as a safety factor.

MOSSEL: Yes, but sometimes this safety mechanism breaks down. Unfortunately, this brings us to the unknown causes of putrefactive diarrhea: combat, a long exposure to high temperatures or reduced temperatures, perhaps psychodynamic factors, etc. One thing is sure: When we detect, in the diarrhea, the typical metabolites of putrefaction they must have been produced.

GUSTAFSSON: That is what I also wanted to emphasize; the fact that under stress conditions and adverse temperature relations, and so forth, you can get these symptoms.

MOSSEL: We know one instance which is purely psychogenic. It stems from our pediatric ward. On the 5th of December we have a national celebration in the Netherlands: Santa Claus, which has nothing to do with your Santa Claus at Christmas time. This involves quite an excitement for the children, because in our ward there will be a Santa Claus visiting with them and handing out sweets. It was a classical phenomenon that the day after Santa Claus there was always an increased amount of diarrhea in the pediatric ward, and the popular interpretation was: Well, the kids eat too many sweets on this occasion.

But then we examined carefully the intake of carbohydrates in these and other periods and found no material differences. This made it likely that "post-Santa Claus gastrointestinal up-sets" were based on a psychomotorically determined disturbance in absorption of normally well-tolerated things, perhaps due to increased peristalsis; for which my colleague, the pediatrician, has introduced the term "psychological resection."

BARNES. When you have diarrhea with proteolytic digestion by bacteria, leading to the production of amines and toxic substances, is there any evidence that there is morphological change in the intestinal wall which leads to an increased absorption of these toxic substances, or are you merely getting an increased production of the amines? Is there any evidence that there is another type of bacterial effect in the sense that there is some inhibition of such detoxifying enzymes as diamineoxidase or monoamineoxidase, or something of this sort?

MOSSEL: Oh, definitely! In the case of the proteolytic diarrhea, which is a protracted diarrhea for a week or a couple of weeks, if you can do a biopsy, as we often do, you will definitely see erosions.

BARNES: But do you think it is this lesion that is leading to the toxicity that is involved?

MOSSEL: We think the lesions are caused by abnormal concentrations of certain bacterial metabolities, such as some amines. When the gut mucosa carries lesions, we have evidence that the monoamineoxidase level in the cells is considerably reduced, so more may get by, and this itself starts a vicious circle, because it now comes into the blood, and it starts the whole thing again.

K. SCHWARZ: Is this established, or is this hypothetical?

MOSSEL: This is established. It will soon be published.

BARNES: I would like to add something that is not established, but is pure speculation. I have thought for a long time that there is a manifestation of toxicity from amines that we consume. Some people are extremely sensitive to beer, for example, and will develop a headache after drinking two or three bottles of beer.

In the same manner certain people are sensitive to wines, and this may well be due to amine-type products which are absorbed, and which might manifest toxicity without any morphological lesion of the intestinal tract, but perhaps a biochemical lesion.

MOSSEL: Well, this may not be so much speculation as you think it is, but there we have no evidence at all.

K. SCHWARZ: I hate to come back to that point, but is it certain that the active compounds are amines, or could these not be other toxins, for instance, endotoxins?

MOSSEL: It could very well be that besides amines other toxic factors are there, but we have rather well precluded endotoxins. We have absolutely precluded staphylo-enterotoxin and endotoxins we have almost certainly excluded also. Let us say, at any rate, it must be metabolites. That is sure.

K. SCHWARZ: It is a basically important point, because we still do not know what makes the necrosis.

MOSSEL: No. We do not know what makes the necrosis in colitis ulcerosa. We find a typical pattern in putrefactive dysbacteriosis, also in colitis nervosa. I would not say this has any causal relationship, but it may be an indication. We believe that the biochemical approach, end-product analysis, to these problems will give us understanding beyond conventional bacteriologic methods.

Dr. Calloway being here, I wonder whether she could give us a brief report about the production of gases, such as methane, in relation to flatulence.

CALLOWAY: Organisms present in the dejecta from well-established ileostomies produce carbon dioxide and hydrogen as the dominant gases, from a variety of substrates, during anaerobic fermentation *in vitro*. The residues from colostomy patients form methane, carbon dioxide and a small amount of hydrogen as well. We have never found an ileostomy sample that produced methane, although it is a regular constituent from colostomy samples. Occasionally, a small amount of acetone is produced.[93]

When intestinal gas is produced in quantity in response to eating a meal that stimulates gas formation, about five to seven hours after the meal there is a rise in breath hydrogen, followed very shortly by a rise in flatus volume and hydrogen content. In most people, methane puddles along in the breath at just about a constant level all day long no matter what test meals are given—quite differently from hydrogen. It behaves as if it were being produced at some level all the time, whereas hydrogen rises and falls.

Not all subjects produce large amounts of methane,[94] so you could get rid of those from your astronaut population, if you wanted to. Preliminary evidence suggests that the population of *Clostridia* is increased in methane-producing subjects.

BROWN: How high does the hydrogen go? I presume it never reaches levels where smoking is dangerous.

CALLOWAY: Oh, 120, 130 parts per million in the breath; but, at usual ventilation rates, that amounts to about 60 or 70 cc. per hour. A good methane producer will have 40 or 50 ppm—as high as 80 parts per million—in the breath all day long.

K. SCHWARZ: How much total methane is that?

CALLOWAY: About 20 to 40 cc. per hour of methane via the lungs. If all you measure is flatus gas, you miss large amounts in many people. Some people ventilate nearly all the hydrogen formed and pass little flatus; others accumulate flatus dominantly.[94]

JENKINS: How about hydrogen sulfide?

CALLOWAY: It is a very small component of flatus, as you know, and we have been looking for what accounts for the volume. We have not studied the minor constituents.

GUSTAFSSON: What about the astronauts? They must swallow oxygen, which is absorbed, so they must have very little gas in their stomach.

RAHN: I would expect it to be very small.

GUSTAFSSON: What about catechols and mercaptans? In a closed system on a long-term flight this might be quite a problem.

CALLOWAY: No doubt about it, but, as I say, everything there at less than 1 percent has not concerned us as yet.

MOSSEL: We have determined quite some amounts of hydrogen sulfide and mercaptans and those things in our cases of proteolytic dysbacteriosis which might, if they occurred in closed environments, be a nuisance.

K. SCHWARZ: They are very toxic. Hydrogen sulfide is more toxic than cyanide.

REYNOLDS: What about higher hydrocarbons?

CALLOWAY: We have used mass and long-path infrared spectrascopy, to examine both flatus and respiratory gases, and have not found anything much longer than 3 or 4 carbons.

REYNOLDS: It would be interesting to see whether these appear in the respiratory or flatus gases of the people in the Sealab, because of the observation that the hydrocarbons produced by bacteria tend to vary directly with pressure.

GUSTAFSSON: So it goes down with reduced pressure?

REYNOLDS: It goes up with increased pressure. Many years ago Zobell demonstrated in oceanic marine bacteria that the chain length of hydrocarbons produced varied directly as the hydrostatic pressure.[95]

That was the reason that I suggested that we study the gases of these people living under high pressure. If the methane in the person were produced by bacteria, you might find that you got ethane as well as methane.

FENN: The organism may change the chain length of the molecules too. *Serratia marinorubra* forms long filaments instead of rods at 600 atm. pressure.[95] They do not divide but they stick together, and thus make long chains, both molecular and organismic.

ARNOLDI: As far as the engineering of the capsule is concerned, there will need to be provision for control of various gaseous contaminants, trace contaminants, such as you mentioned. This does not represent a very large penalty for the environmental control system. The techniques would involve simple adsorption on charcoal, catalytic oxidation, and these represent a minor penalty.

It is a penalty that has to be accepted, though, even if you were to prevent the evolution of these gases from the body, because there is always equipment in the cabin—plastic insulation, and so forth—which will contribute to the same situation.

BARNES: This has not been a problem so far because the capsules to date have been open systems.

ARNOLDI: I was referring to the idealized long-flight system.

GUSTAFSSON: But you have not requested the nutritionists to make diets that are low in the components producing these compounds?

ARNOLDI: It is very desirable to have very small amounts, but in a quantitative sense there is not much difference between a small amount and none.

MUNRO: To what extent do these bacterial attacks on proteins affect the available amino acid supply?

Is this a factor, and is there an improvement in the germfree state in biological value?

CALLOWAY: We have not found any ammonia in gases evolved during anaerobic fermentation *in vitro*—which disturbs us very much. We do find some molecular nitrogen, even though the tubes have been evacuated of air.[93]

BARNES: How much?

CALLOWAY: It depends on the substrate that you use. With some amino acids we may find as much as 8 or 10 percent of nitrogen.

BARNES: Have you tried to calculate to see whether you can solve the problem of the lost 5 percent? *

CALLOWAY: Yes, and I don't think we can. From a mixed substrate, as would be found in the gut, there is higher carbon dioxide production, than with pure amino acids, and very little or no nitrogen is present in the gas formed *in vitro*. At the percentage sometimes found, the tendency would be for nitrogen to enter the gut, not to leave it, because the partial pressure of nitrogen in the blood would be higher than that in the lumen of the bowel. So, if gas is being evolved in volume by bacteria the nitrogen must be in flatus not in the expired air. If the nitrogen present in flatus egested in response to a large meal of beans, for example, actually were produced by the gut flora (and we have no evidence that this is the

* This refers to the amount of dietary nitrogen that is frequently unaccounted by measured losses from the body (in urine and feces) in human nutrition experiments. The magnitude varies with adequacy of methodologic controls. Ed.

case *in vivo*), the loss would still be quite small—in the order of 100 mg., perhaps.

We have not had access to any isotopically-labelled legumes with which we could offer a firm answer—^{15}N-labeled amino acids do not help us because they are readily absorbed high in the small bowel—but we attempted to second-guess the question by measuring ratios of argon to nitrogen in flatus. If the nitrogen were from swallowed air, the ratio should be the same as in atmosphere; if it were evolved, there should be more nitrogen than the argon could account for. We found a bit less, indicating more rapid removal of nitrogen than argon.[99] This might follow from the slower diffusion rate of argon, but also, some of the intestinal anaerobes can fix nitrogen, according to Lorraine Gall.[96] It is much more probable that nitrogen is lost in the form of ammonia than nitrogen gas, in respiration and sweat.

GUSTAFSSON: Depending on the composition of the intestinal microbial flora a fair amount of the protein intake by the host animal is used by the bacteria.

Some types of microorganisms may be digested, so the net outcome would be that the bacterial protein returns to the host protein metabolism. But if the flora mostly consists of bacteria which are not digested by the host, then there is a higher fecal loss of nitrogen, with the voided bacteria.

MUNRO: This will depend, then, on the bacterial types and populations in the upper gut, since in the cecum you would not expect much return.

GUSTAFSSON: Not necessarily if the animal is practicing coprophagy. One must also keep in mind that the small intestine is not sterile which is often postulated. With careful methods you always find bacteria in the stomach and the small intestine. In the lower part of the ileum they are very abundant and very active biochemically. However, we should not let the numbers deceive us, because there are large amounts of bacteria in the large intestine, but most of them are dead, or inactive.

EPSTEIN: Are they bacteria of the usual types in the mouth and colon?

GUSTAFSSON: Yes, although each part of the intestinal tract has a flora, peculiarly its own.

CALLOWAY: I heard not long ago that the organisms that live right in the folds of the mucosa are different from the ones you isolate from the lumen. Is that true?

MOSSEL: That seems to be true, yes. This is almost inaccessible experimentally, because you cannot study this *in vivo* without upsetting something of the normal excretion and neurophysiological feedback. There is almost no approach to that.

GUSTAFSSON: There is a rather recent paper published by Drs. Dubos and Schaedler[97] at the Rockefeller Institute about this, and it is not so much that there are differences in the types of bacteria between the lumen and the wall as in the numbers. Large numbers of lactobacilli are, for example, lodging in the walls of the stomach of mice and cannot be removed by repeated washings.

CALLOWAY: You can enumerate and classify the mucosal inhabitants from the contents just as well as from a biopsy specimen?

GUSTAFSSON: Yes, we believe so, but, on the other hand, it might be that the bacteria most closely associated with the epithelial wall are the most important ones biochemically, because they are in direct contact with the epithelial cells.

MUNRO: Is there any evidence from studies in which a Crosby capsule was used to obtain snippets of mucosa, or is that too crude to give you an index of the bacterial contamination of mucosal villi?

GUSTAFSSON: I believe that there might be changes in the contents of the capsule, including the numbers of bacteria, during the passage of the capsule through the intestinal tract.

I would like to comment on the relation of the diet and the intestinal flora. We have heard that the carbohydrates, of course, influence the composition of the flora. But factors other than dietary could be very effective, in this respect I will give one example. Recently Dick Barnes and others have been putting plastic cups on the tails of rats to prevent coprophagy.

We have used the same technique and examined the contents in the cups, for lactobacilli, and compared the animals which have cups with animals which do not have cups but are fed the same diet. We found (FIGURE 13) that after a certain time there was a decrease in the number of bacteria in the animals not able to practice coprophagy as compared to those who were able to do so. The conclusion would be that there is a need of constant reinfection to keep the flora constant. Dr. Lev[98] has not been able to confirm our findings, but there could be differences in the diet or in the bacteriological technique used in the two laboratories.

I think we must proceed to the next point on the agenda, which concerns what I have termed germfree characteristics. There are many ways to study the relationship between the host animal and the intestinal flora. One of these is to add antibiotics or sulfa drugs to the diet. In this way it is possible to produce vitamin K deficiency, folic acid deficiency, and so forth, which had been difficult before, as these vitamins were made by intestinal bacteria. However, such experiments are sometimes hard to evaluate, because of other effects of the antibiotics.

The best way, maybe, to study these relationships is to raise an animal in completely germfree surroundings from birth on. Although these ani-

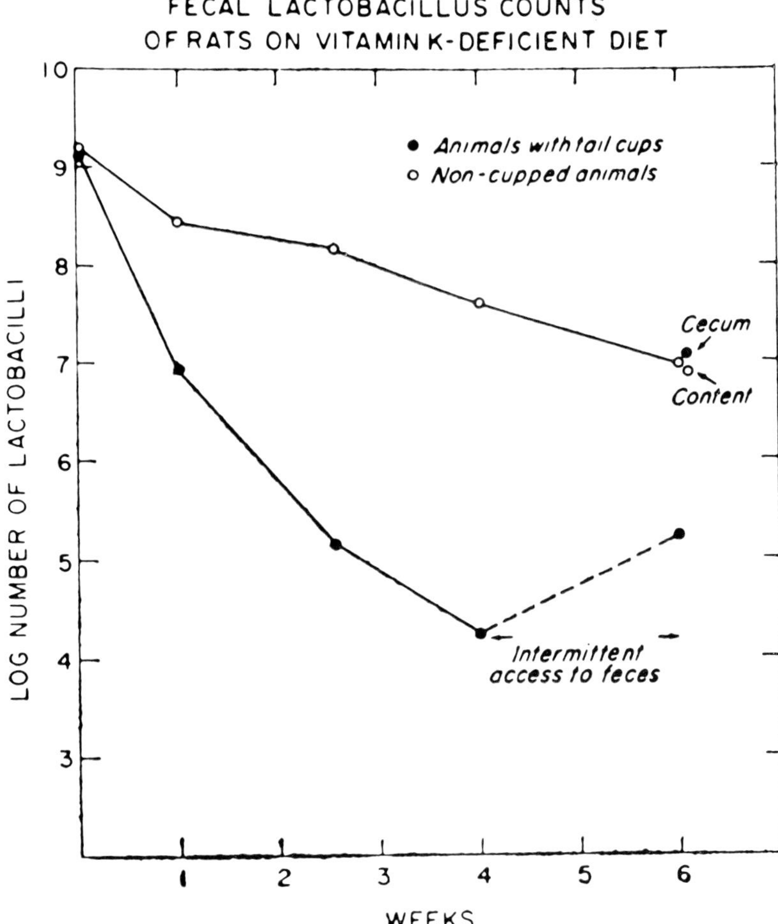

FIGURE 13. Change in fecal flora of animals prevented from practising coprophagy through application of tail cups.

mals might contain viruses, I will in the following refer to them as germfree according to the fact that we find nothing in these animals that grows in our ordinary media.

The rearing of germfree animals involves a series of problems along two lines. The first is how the hardware, *i.e.* the isolators, should be constructed to maintain the animals germfree for years. This includes the principles for the barriers, the sterilization of food, water and air, and the removal of waste. Secondly, all the biological problems concerning the composition of the diet, especially during the lactation period must be taken into account.

The basic principles for the germfree experiments are rather simple and the first successful attempts to raise germfree laboratory animals were published already in 1895. The experiments have until the last few years, however, been of very short duration. It was not until the middle of the 1950's when we were able to get germfree animals to breed inside the isolators that any more detailed studies of the animals *per se* or applied experiments could be undertaken.

POLLARD: May I interrupt a minute? There is a Bibliography of Germfree Research from 1885 to the present,[99] which is available to anyone who requests it from Lobund Laboratory.

GUSTAFSSON: In our laboratory we have been using both stainless steel and plastic jacket isolators. We like the stainless steel better, because they are easier to set up and resterilize, (FIGURE 14). FIGURE 15 demonstrates the last design of the system we use, which is a combined stainless steel and plastic jacket isolator. These are used for large number of animals or when animals are to be kept under conditions that are as close to or the same as the outside as possible. It is literally a room where the attendant is attached to the floor by a suit, which is down into a moat containing a germicidal fluid so she can turn around if she likes to. In this type of isolator we can perform rather complicated experiments.

The large jacket isolator has the same steam autoclave system as the

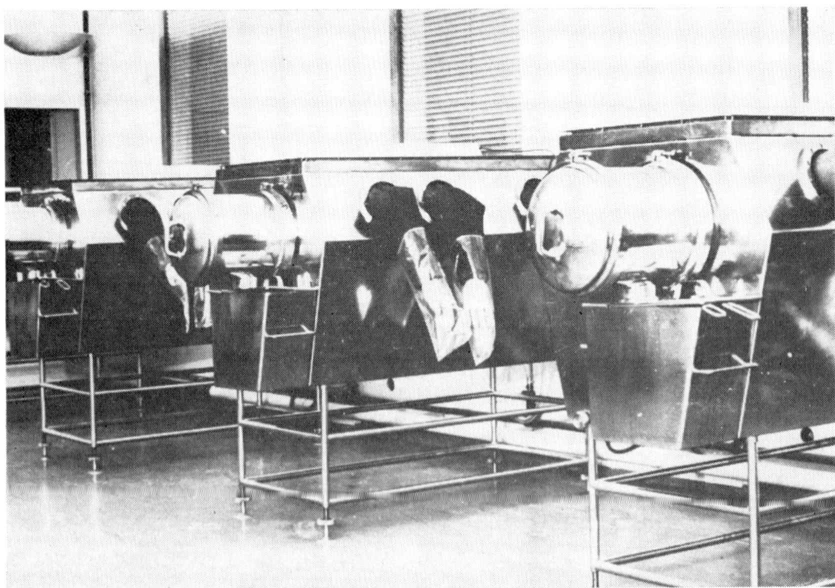

FIGURE 14. Stainless steel isolators for germfree research.

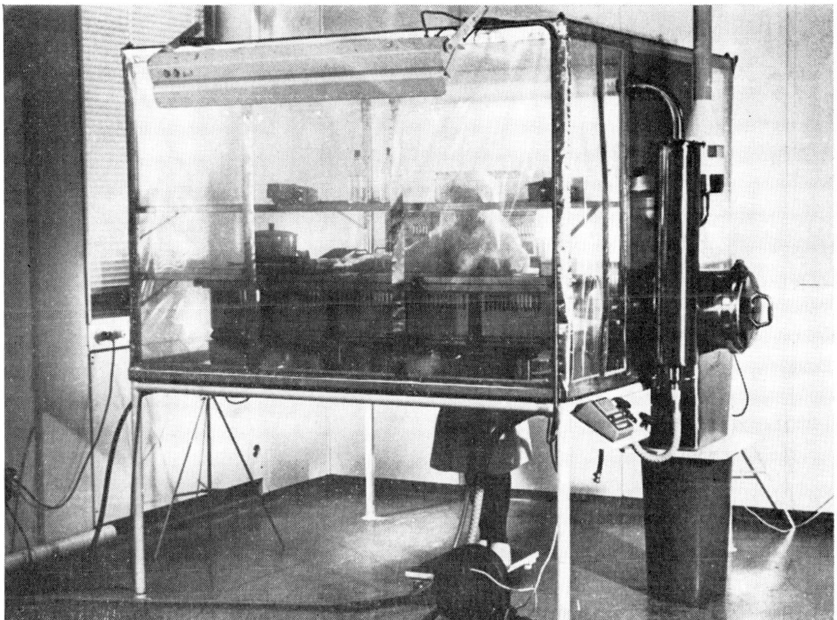

FIGURE 15. Combined stainless steel and plastic jacket isolator.

stainless steel isolators. These autoclaves are used to join two isolators, what some of you would call a docking operation.

Any technique that produces a germfree animal is a good technique, whether it is using plastic or stainless steel isolators. With the help of good technicians there are, nowadays, really very few problems in keeping the animals germfree. Examination of smears from feces and intestinal contents is one of the best ways to test the animal for its freedom from bacteria. In addition to this we are making cultures twice a week using the sterility test methods which are recommended for the control of pharmaceutical products for intravenous administration to patients.

Let us now proceed to the biological problems. How is an animal influenced by the total removal of its so-called normal microbial flora?.

I have already introduced the term germfree characteristics, but when you just look at these animals you cannot tell the difference. They have a nice fur, they grow well as I told before, and there is a breeding that is equivalent to conventional animals. On a semisynthetic diet they have rather soft feces which has no odor. The conditions in a germfree isolator are, however, in many ways peculiar. Food can be kept for months and even a dead animal just dries out.

In TABLE 12 I have noted the composition of the semisynthetic diet we have been using in our germfree rat colony for the past nine years,

TABLE 12

COMPOSITION OF SEMI-SYNTHETIC DIET D7

Casein	22%
Wheat starch	63%
Arachis oil	10%
Salt mixture	4%
Vitamin mixtures	1%
Vitamins added per 100 gm. diet:	
Vitamin A	2100 I.U.
Vitamin D	450 I.U.
Vitamin E	50 mg.
Vitamin K	1 mg.
Thiamine	5 mg.
Riboflavin	2 mg.
Pyridoxine	2 mg.
Calcium pantothenate	10 mg.
Nicotinamide	20 mg.
Choline	200 mg.
Inositol	100 mg.
p-Aminobenzoic acid	30 mg.
Biotin	0.1 mg.
Folic acid	2 mg.
Vitamin B_{12}	0.002 mg.
Ascorbic acid	100 mg.

during which time this colony has reached the 23rd inbred generation. The diet contains a fair amount of ascorbic acid, although the rat does not need that, but we use it as an antioxidant.

K. SCHWARZ: Could I interrupt for a minute? The diet used tends to be deficient in zinc. The Hubbel-Mendel-Wakeman salt mixture was designed before the need for zinc was recognized. The salt mixture is still being sold and used extensively. However, zinc has to be added. I assume that Dr. Gustafsson's animals may get their zinc from the casein. However, there are differences between caseins. If one substitutes an amino acid mixture for the casein in this diet, zinc deficiency will develop. We have seen this inadvertently. It may be the same with manganese.

GUSTAFSSON: We are aware of that, but we have been reluctant to change the diet. We started in 1955, you know, or before that even, and we have done some experiments on other diets with more trace elements added but we find no difference. If we were going to use an amino acid diet, we would of course use another type of salt mixture.

BROBECK: If you leave a dead rat in there, will the other rats eat him?

GUSTAFSSON: No, it has happened only in a few instances.

BROBECK: This is unusual, is it not?

GUSTAFSSON: Our animals are very docile. You can handle them very easily.

POLLARD: It depends on the strain. There are some strains of mice and rats that are quite cannibalistic.

BROBECK: Under these conditions?

POLLARD: Yes. We run into some cannibalism in our animals with tumors, especially when the tumors are eroded and start bleeding.

D. SCHWARZ: Our experience is that rats fed on liquid diets are much more docile than the controls, and this seems to be more or less true of any strain that we have worked with. We have worked with five different strains now.

BROBECK: I think maybe these two things are not related. The ease of handling an animal, and whether it will eat a dead animal might be quite different.

GUSTAFSSON: I will go on, then, with the diet. We had some problems to kill the bacteria in the diet in the beginning but now it can be very easily sterilized and stored. In TABLE 13 I have noted some data on the vitamin content in milligrams per 100 mg. of diet, after autoclaving for 30 minutes at 121 °C.

In order to get a good steam penetration of the powdery diet during autoclaving we mixed the diet with some water and made granules of it. By doing so we in some way or another prevented the oxidation of some diet compounds. The investigators at Notre Dame have very nicely shown afterwards that one gets a better preservation of vitamins up to a certain extent, at least, the more water is added to the diet prior to sterilization.

We have now had our germfree operation running continuously for nine years. We made our last cesarian section in 1956. You have to make cesarian section, of course, to get the first litter and then hand-feed that first litter and hope that they will breed.

The number of accidental contaminations is very low by now. We have about one contamination in a thousand isolator days. By isolator day we

TABLE 13

VITAMIN CONTENT OF DIET D_7 AND AFTER AUTOCLAVING AND STORAGE IN GERMFREE ISOLATOR

Vitamin	Vitamin content mg/100 g diet		
	Freshly made	Autoclaved 30 min 121° C	Autoclaved and stored 30 days
Thiamine HCL	3.9	2.6	1.8
Pyridoxine HCL	1.49	1.35	1.25
Riboflavin	1.70	1.60	1.50

mean, one isolator running for one day, and if ten isolators are running for ten days, that is thus 100 isolator days and so forth.

With the information I have presented so far about our germfree animals you would say that Pasteur's old question, "Is life possible without bacteria?" has been answered in the affirmative. Life is going on in our isolators very well without bacteria.

However, the balance in the germfree animal is very easily upset. During the time 1958–1959 we had a very critical period, because all of our rats came down with a hemorrhagic tendency with a very high mortality, although they had synthetic vitamin K (Menadione) in the diet. We thought, of course, that we had detected a new vitamin-like factor, the equivalent of vitamin K, but it turned out later that the Menadione sulfate we were using was not active in these germfree animals in the dose we had been using, and we had to increase it 100 times to protect these animals.

So we went on and made some studies of vitamin K, as is shown in TABLE 14. All germfree rats on a vitamin K-deficient diet will die sooner or later. The females will live longer, but they will all die within 10 weeks. The conventional rats on the same vitamin K-deficient diet will at the same time be completely normal.

If you feed such a deficient animal a small dose of vitamin K (FIGURE 16) and measure the prothrombin time, it goes up after four hours very dramatically. The other animal which was not dosed stays down at the low deficiency level.

If you take these deficient animals out of the isolators and put them into heavily infected surroundings they go up in prothrombin values very quickly, and after two days they will have attained the normal values (FIGURE 17). If, on the other hand, the deficient exgermfree animals are put in sterilized glass jars in an ordinary laboratory, the prothrombin values stay down all the time, at hemorrhagic levels, which shows that you need the right flora to compensate for this deficiency.

TABLE 14

FREQUENCY OF DEFICIENCY SYMPTOMS IN GERMFREE AND CONTROL ANIMALS ON A VITAMIN K-DEFICIENT DIET

Number of animals	Germfree	Control
Total on diet	44	29
With hypoprothrombinemia	44	0
With bleeding tendency or prothrombin below 10 per cent	42	0
With bleeding tendency	35	0
Dying	12	0

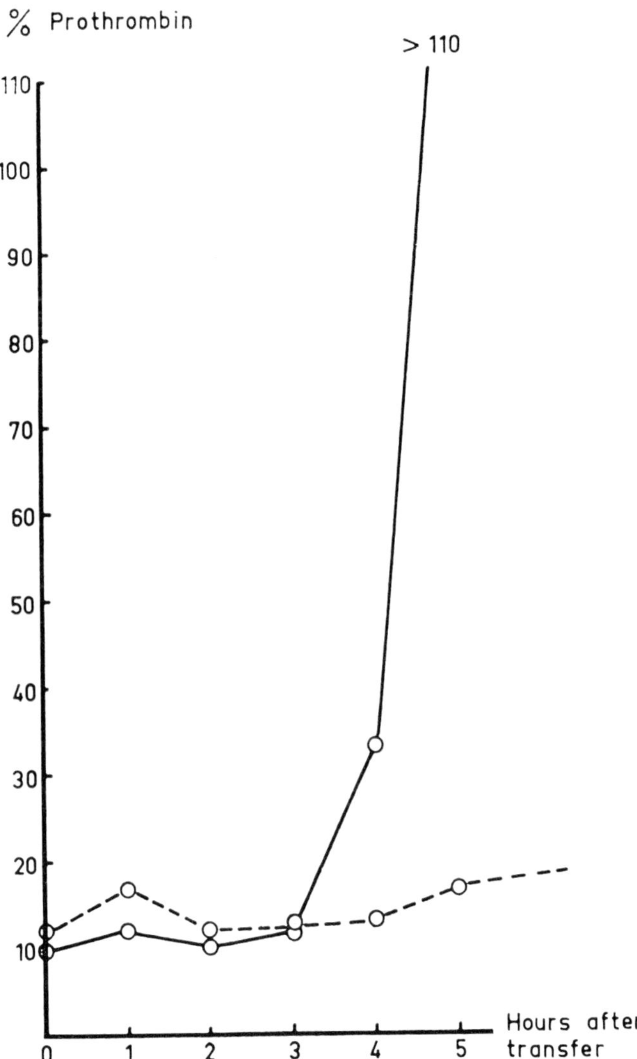

FIGURE 16. Prothrombin values after a single oral dose of 200μg. vitamin K in a germfree rat with vitamin K deficiency (○——○) and of a littermate given sodium chloride solution (○------○) at 0 hours.

We have now come to one of the main points I wanted to make today. That is, not all the bacterial strains of the intestinal tract can compensate for a germfree characteristic like the one we are discussing here. In this case we tested the several microorganisms listed in TABLE 15 for their potency of producing full recovery in these K-deficient rats, but only two

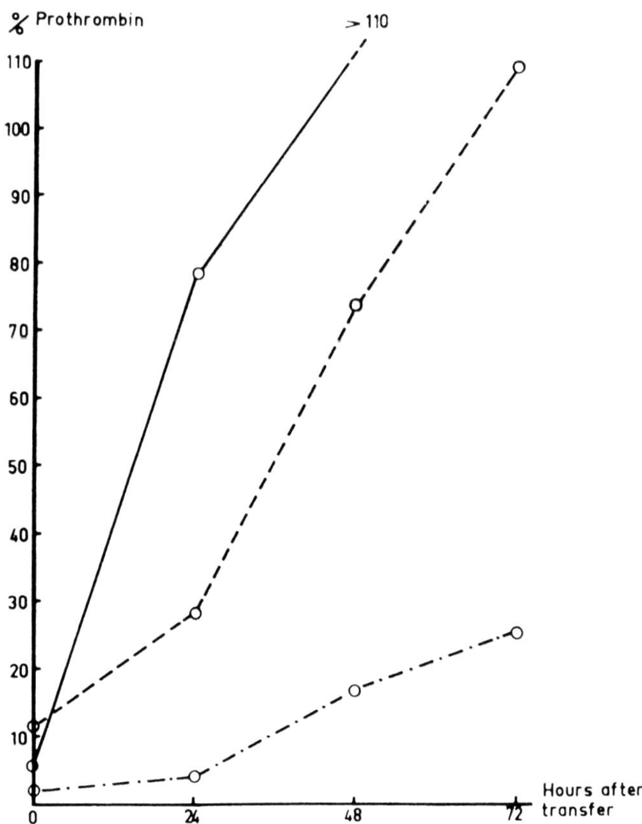

FIGURE 17. Prothrombin values in germfree rats with vitamin K deficiency transferred to a heavily infected ordinary cage (○——○); to a moderately infected metabolism cage (○------○); and isolated in glass jars in the laboratory (○-·-·-·○).

were effective. One of these was an oral strain, which is also found in the intestinal tract. It was very effective—could cure the animals in 24 hours.

Other germfree characteristics are the underdevelopment of the lymphatic organs and the low amount of gammaglobulins. This is the reason for the fact that a high percentage of germfree animals die when transferred to conventional surroundings.

One very obvious characteristic in a germfree rodent is the enlarged cecum (FIGURE 18). The contents are quite different in color from those in the normal animal.

This enlargement of the cecum could be so great that the contents might make up for 10 percent of the body weight, or more. In earlier work in

TABLE 15

EFFECT OF MONOCONTAMINATIONS IN SINGLE VITAMIN K-DEFICIENT GERMFREE RATS

Type of microorganism[1]	Source	48 hours[2] Prothrombin activity values after
		%
Sarcina	rat oral and enteric strain	100
Escherichia Coli	rat enteric strain	100
Lactobacillus acidophilus	rat oral strain	< 10
Diphtheroid	rat oral strain	< 10
Sporeformer	rat enteric strain	< 10
Bacteroides I	rat enteric strain	< 10
Bacteroides II	rat enteric strain	< 10
None	—	< 10

[1] Each animal received the equivalent of 0.1 ml of a 24-hour broth culture which was washed and resuspended in saline.
[2] Initial prothrombin activity < 10%.

this field it was the cause of death of many germfree animals, because the cecum was twisted and a strangulation ileus developed.

Enlarged ceca can also be produced in conventional animals by feeding antibiotics.

FREMONT-SMITH: How did you prevent strangulation ileus in the germfree animals?

GUSTAFSSON: With the diet we are now using the enlargement of the cecum is not maximal, and we very seldom see strangulation.

When the normal intestinal flora is established in the germfree animal there is a rapid reduction of the enlarged cecum. As it is shown in FIGURE 19, it is about 5 percent in the germfree animal but down to the values of the conventional animals, about 1 percent of the body weight, a few days after the contamination. If, on the other hand, a germfree animal is infected with single strains of known bacteria, like proteus, lactobacilli, *E. coli,* nothing happens. So there must be organisms present in the normal intestinal flora which cause a reduction in the cecum in the germfree animal, or, vice versa, in its absence there is enlargement of the cecum. This is not one of the known bacteria. We have had germfree animals infected with up to 15 strains of known bacteria from the intestinal tract in man or in animals, and they still have enlarged ceca.

This means that any of us could have a seemingly normal flora, but we could be lacking this physiologically important organism. We could present symptoms which really belong to the germfree characteristics with a so-called normal flora, because we are lacking this unknown organism. There

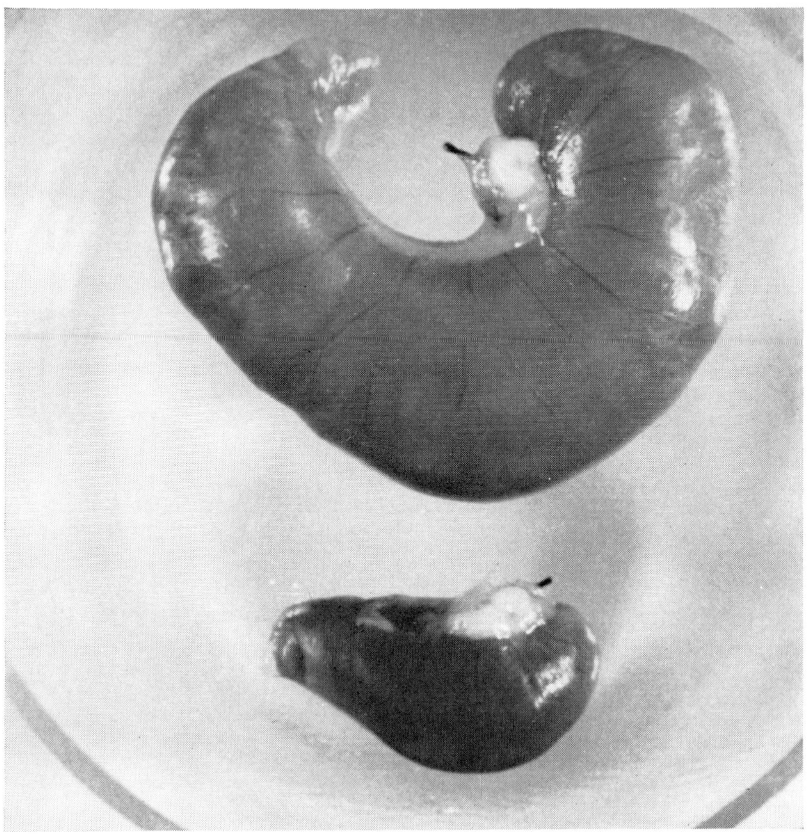

FIGURE 18. Cecum from a male 140 days old germfree rat (top) and from a male 14 days old conventional rat (bottom) reared on the same autoclaved semi-synthetic diet D7.

have been several organisms isolated that have some effect on the cecum, but there has been no one isolated that is fully effective.

What disturbances in the physiology of the cecum are behind this enlargement? This analysis has taken us and several others many years of work, and we do not have the full answer yet. We know, however, that there are several factors involved.

1. It is known that the shedding of the epithelial cells of the intestine of the germfree animal is much slower than in the conventional, which, of course, tends to make the surface of the organ larger and increase its weight.

2. There are reduced motility and reduced sensitivity to some biologically active compound, like acetylcholine.

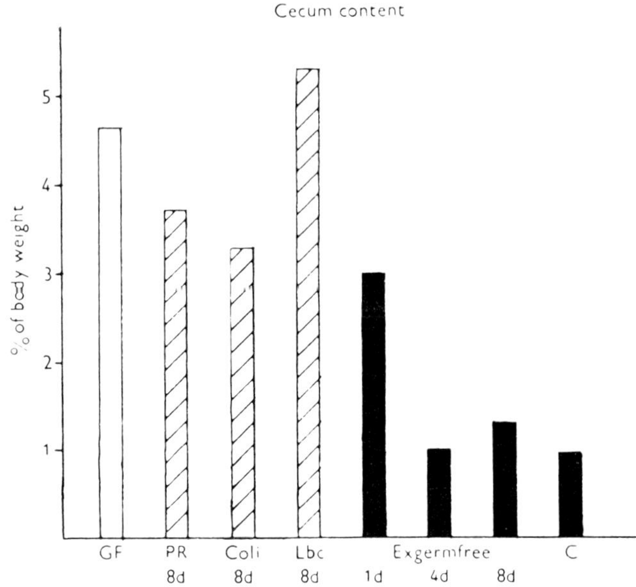

FIGURE 19. The relative weight of the cecum content of germfree and infected rats. Each bar gives the mean of 6–8 animals. GF: Germfree rats. C: Control rats on the same diet. Exgermfree: Germfree rats infected with feces from the control rats. Pr: Germfree rats infected with *Proteus vulgaris*. Coli: Germfree rats infected with *E. coli*. Lbc: Germfree rats infected with *Lactobacillus acidophilus*. 8 d and so forth gives the number of days after contamination.

3. Large amounts of mucin are present in the feces and contents of the large intestine of the germfree rat.

4. There is a high tryptic activity in the feces of germfree rats due to the fact that the normal inactivation of digestive enzymes is impaired.

LIVINGSTON: Has anybody tried the influence of the sympathetics locally? Megacolon in man can be relieved by sympathetic injection with procaine or by sympathectomy. I wonder whether the bacterial influence may be one that affects the autonomic nervous system followed by neuromuscular change, change in sensitivity to drugs, hypersecretion of mucin, and so forth—as secondary results of sympathetic dysfunction?

GUSTAFSSON: It is not hypersecretion of mucin, I think. I think it is a fact that the mucin is not metabolized as it is normally by the intestinal flora.

MOSSEL: Did I understand correctly that the cause of the enlarged cecum is just a stuffing of the interstitial areas with mucin? Is that all that happens on a microscopic scale?

GUSTAFSSON: No, it is the fact that the epithelial cells are not shed at the normal rate. They are kept there, so the epithelial layer is much thicker. The mucin-containing cells, the goblet cells, are there to a higher amount. And the Lieberkühn crypts are not straight. They grow down underneath each other, and the epithelial layer is thicker than it should be.

MUNRO: Have you used tritium to label the nuclei, in order to determine whether the rate of cell transit of the mucosa alters?

GUSTAFSSON: We did not do that, but others did, and there is definitely prolonged lifespan of the epithelial cells.

To continue with the description of the characteristics of the germfree animal, I could go on for the whole afternoon as we have more than 20 listed at present and several new ones are published every year. I think I will end my presentation by briefly mentioning two others, because they demonstrate the added complexity when the presence of several specific microorganisms are necessary. There is no urobilin in the feces of these animals (TABLE 16). When the normal flora was established there was urobilin formed, but it took years to isolate from the conventional flora, the unknown organism that could convert bilirubin to urobilin.

When germfree animals were infected with this organism there was an excretion of urobilins in the feces, but the daily amounts were below those in the conventional animals. When the monoinfected animal was then additionally infected with a strain of *E. coli,* which in itself cannot produce urobilin from bilirubin, the output increased (TABLE 17). This is an example of endosymbiosis, but also of the complexity of interactions, not only with the host but also between the microorganisms.

In germfree animals bile acid is mainly in the form of 7-dehydroxylated compounds. If bile acids labeled with ^{14}C are fed to the animal and recovered daily, one will find that the biological half-life of the bile acid in a conventional rat is about two days, whereas it is about ten days in the germfree rat (FIGURE 20). In the germfree rat feces nothing else but the labeled bile acid is recovered unchanged, whereas in the conventional rats a series of metabolites are found.

The working hypothesis was then that these metabolites were not reabsorbed and entering back into the intrahepatic circulation. This would

TABLE 16

UROBILINS IN FECES FROM GERMFREE AND FROM CONVENTIONAL RATS
Calculated as micromol stercobilinogen per kilogram body weight per 24 hours.

	No. of animals	No. of determinations	Micromol urobilins	
			Mean	Range
Germfree	3	3	0.0	0.0–0.0
Conventional	9	15	3.4	2.1–5.0

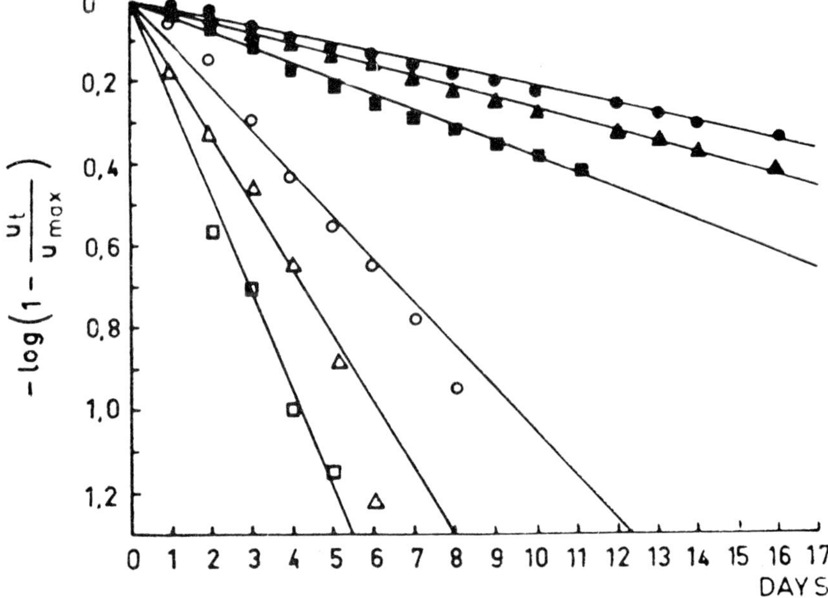

FIGURE 20. Semilogarithmic plot of elimination of cholic acid in conventional (□△○) and germfree rats (■▲●) on the same diet. The half life is 1.2–2.1 days for the conventional and 8–14.5 days for the germfree animals.

be one of the mechanisms by which the body was relieved of the endogenous cholesterol and bile acid. If this was true, these animals should have elevated cholesterol levels—and so they have. On a cholesterol free diet they have elevated cholesterol levels (TABLE 18).

TABLE 17

UROBILINS IN FECES FROM EXGERMFREE RATS CONTAMINATED WITH CLOSTRIDIUM (G 62) OR WITH CLOSTRIDIUM (G 62) + E. COLI (G 14)
Urobilins calculated as micromol stercobilinogen per kilogram body weight per 24 hours.

Animal No.	Contaminated with	Days after contamination					
		3–6	7–10	11–14	15–18	112–115	325
5	*Clostridium* (G 62)	0.12	0.11	0.11	0.34		
6	" "	0.17	0.08	0.11	0.32		
7	" "	0.27	0.15	0.34	0.25	0.72	0.25
8	*Clostridium* (G 62) + *E. Coli* (G 14)	0.52	0.86	0.77	1.34		
9	" "	0.30	0.37	0.91	0.89		
10	" "	0.82	0.79	0.99	0.94		

TABLE 18

SERUM-CHOLESTEROL VALUES IN GERMFREE AND CONTROL ANIMALS

Diet	Group	Number of animals	Serum-cholesterol, *mg. %*		
			Mean	Range	Significance of difference
Standard	Germfree	15	110	189–77	$0.01 > P > 0.001$
	Control	9	77	90–68	
Standard + 0.5% cholesterol	Germfree	17	258	712–97	$P > 0.1$
	Control	14	209	386–107	

As our investigations have proceeded over the years, the complexity of the bile acid metabolism of the intestinal flora has become more and more evident. At least four microorganisms or systems of microorganisms are involved. One is deconjugating, one is 7-dehydroxylating, one is absorbing the metabolites and one is probably cofactor to the others.

All these evidences of an eventual endosymbiosis with microorganisms within the mammalian intestinal tract is interesting, but what has it to do with medicine and what has it to do with space medicine and aeronautics? Well, the answer is very simple: You can have germfree characteristics in so-called normal animals with the so-called normal flora.

Conventional animals that we use are all of the same strain as the germfree animals. From time to time we have been removing germfree animals from the isolators to the animal room, giving them the normal flora, and have kept them there as conventional controls.

When we transferred our laboratory from Lund to Stockholm, we adopted the same procedure and kept these animals in an animal room. We did not, however, infect them with the microbial flora we had in Lund. We let them pick up any kind of microorganisms in Stockholm. After six months they were then examined for some germfree characteristics, listed in FIGURE 21.

In Lund the conventional animals had high amounts of gamma globulin in their sera. In Stockholm the so-called normal animals had rather low amounts of gamma globulin. In Stockholm the so-called conventional animals had active trypsin in the feces. Germfree animals had the same amount of active trypsin in the feces, whereas the conventional ones from Lund had relatively low amounts. The bile acid excretion was in between.

In Stockholm there was not the right symbiotic flora, although the feces of these animals seemed to have a "normal" flora according to ordinary bacteriological methods, including coli, lactobacilli and so on.

As the rats' normal habitat is the soil, it is likely that this also is the source of the endosymbionts in the rats. The situation in the conventional animals in the Stockholm group was also changed, in some respects

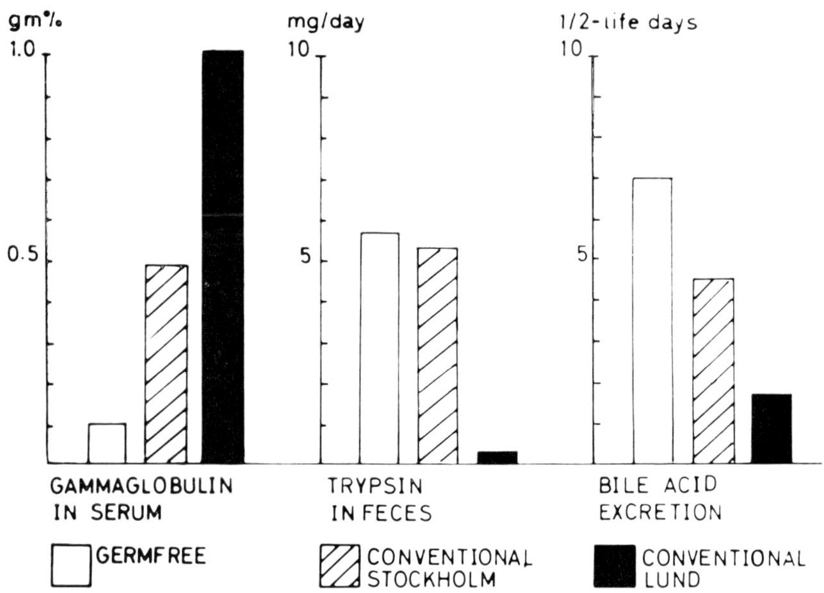

FIGURE 21. Three germfree characteristics—low gammaglobulin content in serum, high trypsin content of feces and slow turnover of bile acids—are retained in conventional animals reared in isolated animal rooms (conventional Stockholm) as compared to animals of the same strain in open rooms (conventional Lund).

equal to that in the Lund group, when the rats were fed different soil specimens.

I have demonstrated that the germfree animals show a series of symptoms or characteristics which normally are counteracted or compensated by the presence of microorganisms which you could very well label symbiotic. Symbiotic microorganisms isolated thus far are typically anaerobic, and not easily cultured or classified. When all the symbionts have been classified they should counteract all the germfree characteristics when established in a germfree animal as the *minimal necessary flora.* My presentation has also suggested that such germfree characteristics may occur in an host organism with an intestinal flora that would be labeled normal with our ordinary bacteriological diagnostic methods.

Now, what is the likelihood that we should get a change in the intestinal flora with the possible loss of symbionts in a closed system like a space capsule? Has somebody had any experience along these lines?

We have kept animals for a long time in these isolators with a minimal and well defined flora of six bacterial strains and no flora change has happened so far, but we did not have any increased oxygen tension, and we did not put them into a stress situation.

I would also like to point out that if you lose one of these symbiotic bacteria in a closed system, you can never get it back. If an astronaut is dependent on one of his endosymbionts and he loses that, he cannot get it back.

FREMONT-SMITH: Except from another astronaut.

GUSTAFSSON: Yes. If you know which these are, you could keep cultures of them freeze-dried and feed them to the astronauts. That, of course, is only in a situation when you know which the endosymbionts are.

Another factor that is very important has to do with Dr. Mossel's presentation. If the astronaut gets a *Staphylococcus aureus* over-growth, for example, he would get in serious trouble. That is why I started out with this very provocative statement that the intestinal flora might be one of the most dangerous things that he is carrying with him. The only part that is lacking in my chain of reasoning is evidence: How often do we get the flora drift in a man confined in an area like the space ship? I very strongly suggest that when you do experiments in closed systems, the intestinal flora should be very closely followed.

WARD: I should comment on your suggestion that space simulator studies include bacteriological studies. Most of the simulator work at the USAF School of Aerospace Medicine at Brooks Air Force Base has been supported by very active bacteriological programs.

GUSTAFSSON: I know, but they have been using standard methods looking for the known bacteria strains only.

WARD: They have been using standard methods, true, but they have not found significant shifts in intestinal flora.* They may be overlooking a few organisms, perhaps quite a few, but the population sampled is still large.

Dr. James E. Moyer is responsible for most of the Air Force work. He has an active, well-planned bacteriological program going, and has published his findings.[100]

GUSTAFSSON: But, what we are suggesting Dr. Mossel and myself—is another thing. If you incubate a feces sample from a person with ^{14}C-labeled bile acid and then follow the metabolites in the fecal suspension, you can tell whether the right microorganisms are there. You should study the metabolites, not the bacteria.

---

* A recent report indicates that there is a shift in predominant anaerobic bacteria associated with consumption of a space-type diet. See P. E. Riely et al., *Aerospace Med.,* p. 820, Aug. 1966. Ed.

You could also test the trypsin content. You should test the hexosamine output, and so on. Do not care too much about the bacteria because many of them die in the bacteriologist's culture media. There is a tremendous amount of bacteria that neither Mossel, myself nor any other bacteriologist can get to grow in pure cultures.

REYNOLDS: Do you recommend minimal intestinal flora, as compared with the complete gamut of normal flora for an astronaut? In other words, would you establish a specific flora and delete *Staph. aureus,* for example?

GUSTAFSSON: In a way I would prefer to have the astronauts completely germfree. As one cannot use running water or vacuum cleaners in a germfree isolator, they are hard to keep clean in experiments running for a year or more. Fecal material, food and so forth has to be handled with the same gloves and there is a tendency in that all this is distributed over the surfaces of the interior of the isolators. This is of very little trouble in the germfree state where there are no microorganisms to cause any decay of this organic material. In a germfree spacecraft many problems concerning personal hygiene, food storage and waste disposal should be easy to solve.

In an isolator with *conventional* animals, the difficulties with cleaning poses a major problem, especially if the humidity is high. Mold grows everywhere, on the diet, in the cages and so on. As these animals very often have diarrhea this constant ingestion of molds is undoubtedly interfering with the animals' general condition. I might have too much of an imagination, but sometimes I think that these isolators with the conventional animals, smelling badly and filled with mold and mold spores, would reflect the situation in a space craft on a long-term mission, when people get tired of cleaning up.

The germfree state is not the ideal either, because there is always the problem of the germfree characteristics. Some of these we have been able to compensate with a minimal flora, as we define it at present. These animals have been kept for months without losing any of this set of bacteria.

REYNOLDS: Do you think it is possible to make astronauts germfree and put them in a spacecraft which is completely germfree and maintain them germfree for an entire three-year flight?

GUSTAFSSON: If you could get them germfree, sterilize the capsule, and get them in there, it would be very easy to keep it sterile. This I might say is not impossible to do.

KRAUSS: Have these experiments ever been run with germfree humans?

GUSTAFSSON: No, but experiments are going on in order to sterilize an adult conventional animal and make it germfree. I must tell you how it is done.

The animal is for three days given a cocktail of antibiotics, and then one lets it dive through a germicide, into a sterilized isolator. It is then kept in this isolator for three days and given another three days of antibiotic treatment and a new dive into a new isolator. Each time this is repeated the bacterial flora is considerably reduced.

BARNES: Dr. Levenson in the Department of Surgery at Albert Einstein College of Medicine has been keeping under germfree conditions, human beings who have been badly burned.* How close has he gotten to the establishment of a germfree human?

GUSTAFSSON: If you sterilize the room—the food—and give the patients a treatment of antibiotics—both local and general, the flora is reduced both from a quantitative and qualitative point of view.

You will say: Well, the skin is infected, and it must reinfect itself all the time. But it does not, and we cannot explain why. My suggestion is that this is a situation where the numbers of bacteria come below a certain level where they cannot, so to say, survive any more, and this is a well-known bacteriological phonomenon.

MOSSEL: Pasteur Effect No. 1.

K. SCHWARZ: Would not the hypothetical germfree human in many ways be a completely abnormal human being? How do you know whether this would be a desirable situation?

I think from the fact that this human would not be able to metabolize bile acids, cholesterol and many other constituents as effectively as under conventional conditions, or to do a lot of other things which happen due to the symbiosis with microorganisms in the GI tract—he may not be able to fulfill his function, or his mission.

What do you know about germfree animals and stress, for one thing? What are their adrenals like? How do they operate psychologically? Would not all these questions have to be answered before one can make a statement of that sort?

GUSTAFSSON: Yes. My statement was intended to be provocative, and, I must say, I would hope not to be in the position to send a germfree man away somewhere; but if you draw the conclusions of the present situation in our field, it is easier to handle the germfree animal than the conventional animal, if you want a defined and controlled situation from a microbial point of view.

ARNOLDI: Does the docility of the germfree animal have any implications with regard to the possible mental state of the human being?

FREMONT-SMITH: Would the humans be gentle too?

ARNOLDI: I do not care whether he is gentle. Maybe he has lost the capacity to react to a difficult situation.

* Personal communication.

GUSTAFSSON: Please, do not take it for granted that the germfree animal is more docile than the conventional one because we have not made any objective tests on that. This is just an impression we have. It should not be quoted as a scientific finding or something like that. You heard Dr. Pollard say that he had just the reversed impression.

But on the positive side, the germfree animal seems to have a longer lifespan than the conventional one, although we have not made any large-scale investigation into this with large number of animals.

FREMONT-SMITH: How much is the lifespan increased, in percentage?

GUSTAFSSON: It depends on what you compare with. The maximum lifespan in our germfree rats is three-and-a-half years.

FREMONT-SMITH: This is a germfree three-and-a-half years?

GUSTAFSSON: Yes, under ordinary open animal room conditions they might not live more than one-and-a-half years, but in our SPF* colony they live two-and-a-half to three years. So I think the net result is about a half-a-year lifespan prolonagtion.

This agrees rather well with your experience does it not Dr. Pollard?

POLLARD: Yes, we have had several colonies that went over three-and-a-half years. We had to terminate our experiment so we do not know how long ours would have lasted. Strangely, the survival ratio of males to females was reversed over that of the conventionals. There were more males surviving than females. Most of the deaths in aging germfree animals were degenerative in nature: obstructive lesions, glomerulonephritis, cardiovascular diseases, and pulmonary diseases.

REYNOLDS: I would like to press Dr. Gustafsson to answer the original question, concerning a comparison between a controlled human flora as compared with a conventional uncontrolled one.

GUSTAFSSON: I would say that if we knew how the necessary minimal microbial flora should be composed that would be the best to establish.

REYNOLDS: In other words, we should be trying to find out as fast as we can what those symbionts are, if possible. Is that right?

GUSTAFSSON: Yes.

JENKINS: There is more or less of an ecological dictum that a multiplicity of species gives you stability. If you pick out specific ones and have just a few in any culture, these go up and down. If you have just a few species, and you cannot control the culture, you have wide variability.

The idea of a defined, limited flora is extremely attractive, but I am inherently afraid of it.

---

* SPF = Specific-Pathogen-Free

VI. REGENERATIVE SYSTEMS REEXAMINED*

Discussion Leader:

DALE JENKINS
Bioscience Programs
Office of Space Science and Applications
National Aeronautics and Space Administration
Washington, D.C.

JENKINS: The first method of environmental control used in the Mercury, Gemini and Apollo programs, is just to carry along the required oxygen and food. A means is provided for removing carbon dioxide and recirculating some of the air. The present system also permits wastage; the leak rate, for example, in Wally Schirra's Mercury capsule was 688 cc. per minute.

In the future, it will be necessary to button the capsules up as tightly as possible. We can go into partial or nearly complete regenerative systems, using chemical or bioregenerative methods.

The term "bioregenerative system" indicates that organisms are used for regeneration. This can provide for both atmosphere and food. However, I am avoiding the term "closed ecological cycle" because this means that you have a completely sealed unit where everything is used, recirculated, and so on. This is a very nice ultimate goal, but a very difficult one to achieve. In the Hydrogenomonas system as presently conceived, for example, we throw away the feces. In the algal system it may be possible to utilize everything.

After the trip to the moon in 1970, or at about this period, we may have manned orbiting laboratories. Some of these may be up for a year or more, and these will probably have at least a chemical regenerative system, even though resupply is planned. Some of the larger craft—with many men, for longer periods of time—may have more advanced regenerative systems.

However, the first truly regenerative system that would be required, probably, would be for the planned manned Martian mission, somewhere

* For additional discussion, see Volume I of this series.

in the neighborhood of 1980. This mission will probably involve six to ten men, and might take three years. With such a mission there would *have* to be greater regenerative efficiency, unless we have more effective and efficient propulsion systems than we are presently anticipating.

It would take on the order of a quarter of a million pounds—about 100,000 kg.—of material to support ten men for three years. It would take about 6,000 cubic feet, if all of the oxygen and food were stored, and all of the waste products—CO_2 and so on—were to be stored.

The chemical regenerative systems are perhaps farther along then the biological systems. However, there is still a great deal to be done, and the real expense is ahead of us. When you get into engineering scale-up and development of pilot plants, then you get into real money. I think it is essential that in the very near future the various agencies concerned, and their advisers, get together and decide which system is the better candidate for development or determine whether more than one system is necessary. There is also a question whether the regenerative life support systems can be made to work at the level at which it is possible to fund them and in the time involved.

Chemical Systems of Atmosphere Regeneration

ARNOLDI: Let me describe four different phases, or classes, of space flight, which in one sense may be evolutionary developments—technical evolution—but in another sense may actually be four different requirements for four different types of vehicles and systems.

I will describe the four phases in terms of the most salient characteristics (FIGURE 22). One obvious characteristic that needs to be considered is duration—duration of unresupplied missions. Phase I is up to two weeks. This would be typical of Mercury, Gemini, the earlier Apollo flights. Phase II—and I'll explain later why this is true—is one to eight weeks.

PHASE	I	II	III	IV
DURATION	TO 2 WEEKS	1–8 WEEKS	1–12 MONTHS	YEARS
POWER SOURCE	CHEMICAL	← SOLAR OR NUCLEAR →		
POWER PENALTY	LB/KW–HR (>.5)	← LB/KW → 200	50	20?
WATER	STORED	RECLAIM	RECLAIM	INTEGRATED SYSTEMS
OXYGEN	STORED	STORED	RECLAIM	
CO_2	ABSORB	DISPOSE	DECOMPOSE	
FOOD & WASTES	STORED	STORED	STORED	

FIGURE 22. Essential characteristics of space missions.

Phase III is one to twelve months, and Phase IV I will just say is years, not specifying how many years.

I have arbitrarily listed a number of facts which are pertinent to the description of the four phases of flight. One is the nature of the power source—not propulsive power, but secondary power for making use of the abilities of the people and the equipment involved in the mission. Phase I will be chemical power, meaning batteries or fuel cells. (Fuel cells are batteries, so I make no distinction there.) Phases II, III, and IV will be solar or nuclear sources of energy, which means that the energy can be converted to electric power, involving some sort of vapor cycle heat engine and an electric generator.

The penalty paid for the use of electric power is significant to the evaluation of the logistics problems of the various systems planned. I will not even specify what the power penalty is numerically in Phase I, but the important thing is that the units of it are pounds per kilowatt hour. In general that number will be something much greater than 0.5.

Phases II, III, and IV would be characterized by power penalties measured in pounds per kilowatt. In other words, they are systems which transform or generate energy without the degradation of their own material and can operate indefinitely without the necessity for using expendable material. The typical number would be, I propose, 200 pounds per kilowatt for Phase II, which is something which would be feasible with present concepts of solar power generation—not solar cells. (They would be heavier than this.) It might be possible with nuclear power with a fairly heavy amount of shielding, and of course in both cases it depends critically upon the size of the installation.

Phase III represents an advance in the state of the art, probably in the direction of achieving lighter weights of shielding for nuclear systems, and might achieve 50 lb. per kilowatt.

Phase IV, the ultimate, really—I think I am conservative in saying that 20 lb. per kilowatt would be an interesting target, but there is some question as to whether it could be achieved.

These base figures critically determine the kind of systems we can consider for the several phases, and are very strict requirements for the development of the state of the art for each of the subsystems powered by this electrical source.

Let us consider some of the vital aspects of life support. Obviously, the first one is oxygen supply; The Phase I system involves stored oxygen and this is proposed also in Phase II. In Phase III we may, because of the possibility of more sophisticated reclamation systems, be able to regenerate oxygen from carbon dioxide and water.

Water, as a second requirement, would be stored in Phases I and II; in Phase III, it would be reclaimed from urine or other liquid wastes.

CO_2 would be absorbed by chemisorbents in Phase I, such as lithium hydroxide, as used in current missions. In Phase II it would be disposed overboard. In Phase III we may decompose and dispose of the carbon from the CO_2.

The fourth major topic is food and wastes. These are stored for Phases I, II, and III—the latter may be debatable.

Phase IV is the opportunity for the algal systems and other fairly sophisticated bioregenerative systems. Let us just say that the water, oxygen, CO_2, and food problems are denoted by an integration of systems. If we are truly to achieve a closed ecology, which, I agree with Dr. Jenkins, is a will-o'-the-wisp of the very far future, that would represent a full integration of these functions, plus other functions.

Some compromises may be made, and I would tentatively suggest that the bioregenerative systems mentioned here would come into being somewhere on the fringes of Phase III and Phase IV. I do not want to slice it too fine, but I do believe that the chemically regenerative systems represent perhaps the earlier stages of Phase III, and how far they go depends upon the relative state of the art at the time that particular missions are devised and implemented.

My purpose here is to provide a framework against which we can consider and define the nature of various subsystems. There is some overlapping of phases because of the uncertainty of the figures involved, and because I have not spelled out specific missions.

For example, Apollo could just as well be a Phase II mission, if it had a different kind of power supply. It is the choice of power supply, which is a matter of expedience rather than pure logic, which has resulted in Apollo being classified in Phase I in my terminology. Actually, Apollo could be made a Phase II project even with a chemical power source, which would be on the basis of a high-grade chemical power source (such as hydrogen–oxygen fuel cells), employed with a CO_2 removal system which dumps the CO_2 overboard into space, which turns out to be competitive weightwise with lithium hydroxide for a two-week mission. The decision has been made—rightly, I think—by NASA to use lithium hydroxide for Apollo, in accordance with the available state of the art, without requiring exotic hardware, but I think somewhat further in the future an Apollo-type mission would be undertaken under Phase II rather than Phase I.

KRAUSS: Could you just very briefly mention what type of solar power systems you have in mind for Phases II, III, and IV?

ARNOLDI: I am talking about a category of systems, rather than particular devices. Solar energy electric systems are feasible, primarily in terms of using a closed vapor cycle heat engine in order to convert the received energy into mechanical power, to drive an electric generator.

You can consider exotic—I will call them exotic systems even when they exist, such as solar cells—systems which directly convert solar energy to electrical energy, but they are rather heavy, and they are not going to be within the category of power penalties that we are considering here.

This does not matter very much if you only need 50 watts per satellite, but when you want 100 kilowatts this becomes a different matter. You need a football-field size of solar cell array, and you need box cars to carry power, which turn out to be rather weighty if you are talking about Phases III and IV.

In order to achieve a low power penalty it is necessary to have a system which collects and concentrates solar energy before conversion into some other form of energy, to convert this solar energy to a thermodynamic cycle, and then to electrical energy, so that we concentrate the massive parts of the equipment in a unique location, rather than spread them out over a large collection area.

MUNRO: These separations into phases, of course, will be more complicated, because the objective is not merely travel but also work outside the capsule, and therefore it may not be possible to predict an unmixed system. In other words, you will have to allow for periods during which the astronaut will be separated from his capsule, and therefore will have to employ a different system.

ARNOLDI: The characterization of any particular vehicle system into one of these phases gets very cloudy when you get into practical matters. For example, I could crudely say that Phase I ultimately would represent the earth-to-orbit ferry, the resupply vehicle for an orbital satellite, for example. Phase II might represent the occasionally resupplied satellite, perhaps on a resupply period of one to eight weeks. Phase III might be the lunar base that gets resupplied every six months or more. Phase IV might perhaps be a colony on Mars, assuming that it cannot be based on natural resources of the planet.

However, if the resupply problem of Phase II, the orbital satellite laboratory, for example, involves questions of economics or logistics such that it is desirable to have a resupply mission every month in order to change the crew, just because people go stir crazy, or something of that sort—but at the same time we decide we cannot afford it in the national budget to keep on resupplying inorganic materials or foods, and so forth—we may actually want to operate an ecology in Phase III, but with a resupply frequency characteristic of Phase II.

This makes things a little bit more confusing and involves a complexity of tradeoffs among the various considerations.

BROBECK: Could I ask a very simple question? What is the temperature of the outside of the capsule on the side toward the sun?

ARNOLDI: I cannot define it as generality. It depends upon the characteristics of the material, upon the heat flux absorbed by the material, and also its ability to radiate. The surface coating of the Gemini capsule has been chosen to have a reasonable base level of temperature where the internal environmental control system, which involves cooling by means of water evaporation, has essentially a vernier job to do, where it does not have to bear the whole problem of rejecting heat.

FREMONT-SMITH: Will it not vary from the surface which is exposed to the sun to the surface which is in the shade?

ARNOLDI: Right, and therefore a system of either systematic or random rotation or change in orientation is desirable.

FREMONT-SMITH: And also the day and night situation, when it is going around the earth.

ARNOLDI: The whole capsule is so massive that an hour-and-a-half orbital situation does not cause any highly significant effects, so far as the required capacity of the environmental control system is concerned.

BROBECK: What are the extremes? What kind of a gradient can you count on—that is, for using a heat pump, or something like that, between the two sides of the capsule?

ARNOLDI: If you want to use a heat pump, the question is: At what temperature need the condensing side of the heat pump be operating? You can reject heat at temperatures as high as 250°F.

BROBECK: Suppose you want to use the capsule itself as the source of heat and as a deep freeze. What temperatures will you have on the freezing side, and on the hot side?

ARNOLDI: Under equilibrium conditions you could achieve, by using proper coatings on the capsule, temperatures in excess of 200°F, and probably lower than −40°F.

This is critically dependent upon the nature of surface coatings, but the important thing is that on the hot side the amount of energy is limited ultimately by the solar flux, something like 125 watts per square foot, as I recall, and that is not very much energy.

K. SCHWARZ: How much does that decline as you go away and get to Mars?

ARNOLDI: As the square of the distance.

K. SCHWARZ: That must be a terrific loss, then, if you want to have a solar system for the power source.

ARNOLDI: The solar system is not then very attractive. I was not recommending it. I was saying that it was eligible, assuming earth-orbital conditions. Certainly, if you want to go to Mars or Jupiter or further, solar energy is out of the picture completely. For the long run I certainly favor nuclear power sources, particularly to provide flexibility of mission objectives.

TAPPEL: What is the rationale of storing the wastes for such long periods of time?

ARNOLDI: "Storing" is a word which is commonly used to include the notion of throwing it overboard. "Stored" means that it is no longer available for use.

MAYER: It comes along with you even if you throw it overboard.

LIVINGSTON: When you slow down to land on a planet all the stuff you have been ejecting will plaster itself on the planet ahead of you.

BROWN: It is not entirely a joke. This is at the moment an operational decision for NASA with regard to the Apollo mission.

ARNOLDI: It may get out of phase with you. It will certainly have a similar orbit, and the period of the orbit may be almost the same, but with the slightest orbital deviation due to the process of throwing, the phasing will very rarely come out the same, so that the nearest approach in the next opposition may be several miles apart.

Next I was going to try to outline some CO_2 and oxygen reclamation systems in connection with this concept of phases of space flight.

For Phase I, which is Mercury, Gemini, or Apollo, lithium hydroxide was the preferred technique for CO_2 control. This represents a system in which there is a chemical reaction, lithium hydroxide plus CO_2 giving lithium carbonate plus water.

The weight of CO_2 that is to be absorbed by the lithium hydroxide is determined by the stoichiometry of the equation shown in FIGURE 23.

PHASE I — $2LiOH + CO_2 \rightarrow Li_2CO_3 + H_2O$

PHASE II — REGENERABLE SOLID ADSORBENTS
FREEZE–OUT
SEMI–PERMEABLE MEMBRANES
ION EXCHANGE RESINS

PHASE III — SABATIER $CO_2 + 4\,H_2 \rightarrow CH_4 + 2\,H_2O$

BOSCH $CO_2 + 2\,H_2 \rightarrow C + 2\,H_2O$

FUSED Li_2CO_3 ELECTROLYSIS | $Li_2CO_3 \rightarrow Li_2O + C + O_2$
| $CO_2 \rightarrow Li_2O + Li_2CO_3$

SOLID ELECTROLYTE | $CO_2 \rightarrow CO + O$
| $2\,CO \rightarrow C + CO_2$

PHASES III & IV — BIO–REGENERATIVE SYSTEMS
ALGAL SYSTEMS

FIGURE 23. Carbon dioxide control system principles.

In practice the entire contents of the lithium hydroxide canister cannot be fully utilized if we are going to maintain an acceptable CO_2 partial pressure in the output gases. So that, where there is roughly a one-to-one ratio between mass of hydroxide required for mass of CO_2, in practice you may have to have as much as two pounds of lithium hydroxide per pound of CO_2 depending upon the technical economics of the engineering design problem. So, in Phase I the CO_2 is not only stored, but it is stored with an equal or greater weight of lithium hydroxide, which serves no other purpose.

However, it takes only a small amount of fan power to recirculate cabin air through a canister of lithium hydroxide. Therefore, in a system where the power penalty is large, where you have to pay for your power performance of the system in pounds per kilowatt hour, this becomes a reasonable compromise system.

In Phase II we get a little bit more sophisticated, and consider regenerable solid absorbents, freezing, semipermeable membranes, ion exchange —these are the four methods most likely to be given serious consideration for a Phase II type of mission.

The first of these four, regenerable solid absorbents, represents a fully-developed system and it is being used right now in earthside laboratory experimentation. It could be qualified for space flights any time somebody chose to. As of right now there is no defined mission that would require it, although it is anticipated that there will be in the future. The other systems—freezing, semipermeable membranes, and ion exchange resins —have all been given considerable study and have been rejected temporarily for early Phase II missions on the basis of excessive power requirements. This attitude could change considerably if we could get down to 100 lb. per kilowatt.

"Regenerable solid absorbents" designates a system in which a molecular sieve—a regenerable absorbent for CO_2—is used selectively to remove CO_2 from the recirculated atmosphere. The desorption of the molecular sieve is accomplished by exposure to vacuum—to space vacuum —whereby CO_2 is dumped overboard.

BROWN: What about the water?

ARNOLDI: Water becomes a major problem in this system; in fact, because molecular sieves have a preferential affinity for water, and, because the absorption of water then precludes the possibility of absorbing CO_2 it is necessary to predry the air that is processed through the molecular sieve. The technique is to have a pair of silica gel canisters which are cyclically operated from a source of cabin air (see FIGURE 24). Air is brought in through a fan, cyclically through one silica gel canister, and the other. The output from either canister, then, is valved to a distribution

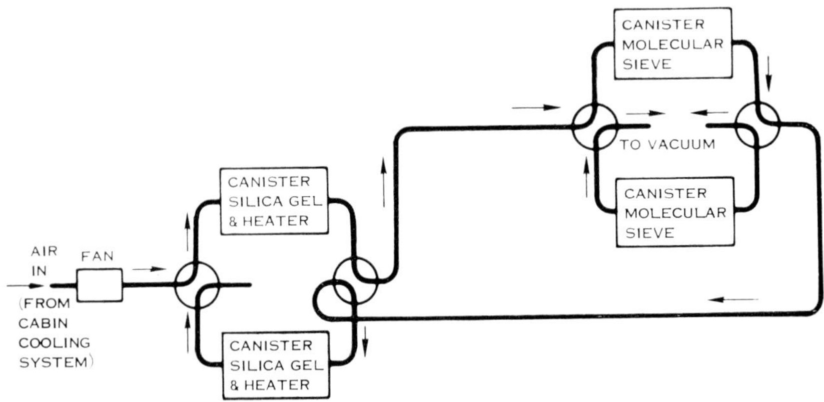

FIGURE 24. Regenerable solid adsorbent system for CO_2 separation.

system which involves two molecular sieve canisters which can be vented to vacuum or can return air to the other side of the silica gel system.

FIGURE 24 shows a basic system in which cabin air is processed by sending it through a silica gel canister where the moisture content is reduced to 5 or 10 parts per million; in other words, near $-100°F$ dew point. The dried air continues on to a molecular sieve canister, which removes CO_2. Generally if we have a half percent CO_2 coming into the system, by means of a molecular sieve we can control the average level of CO_2 leaving the system to less than a tenth of one percent.

From this molecular sieve canister the air returns to the center and is diverted to the second silica gel canister, which has previously been loaded with moisture, and which is now heated by electrical heaters, so that the CO_2-free air is able to pick up the moisture and be rehumidified thereby, and conserve the moisture, which is thereby returned to the cabin.

After the first silica gel canister is loaded with moisture, when it is no longer able to perform its desiccant function, then we have to switch this system so that the incoming air goes through the opposite silica gel canister, which has been revived by the desorption which takes place while the CO_2-free air is going through it. The same occurs in the molecular sieve canisters. While one canister is being used to pick up CO_2 the other one is being discharged into space.

The whole thing can be packaged into a weight of about 65 lb. for three men, with an average power requirement of 300 watts continuous.

The freezeout system involves using either a supplementary fluid or the processed air as the refrigerant, to bring the temperature down to a level where CO_2 can be removed as a solid. In other words, you have to get down to temperatures below -200°F, despite the common knowledge of the freezing point of CO_2 being -109°F. This is, of course, only true at atmospheric pressure, and the saturation temperature drops as we lower the partial pressure.

The freezeout system becomes a rather complex plumbing arrangement. In order to achieve low enough temperatures for freezeout, the heat pumping function is rather demanding of power in terms of known performance of eligible equipment. So it's possibilities are some time in the future, but not for early missions in Phase II.

By semipermeable membranes, I am referring to the concept of separating CO_2 by progressive enrichment through a cascaded series of membranes, possibly silicone rubber, each of which preferentially passes CO_2 by comparison with oxygen or nitrogen. Air enters one side of a device separated into two parts by a membrane and in the passage to the side of lower pressure loses some of its CO_2 (see FIGURE 25). This low-pressure air could go through a compressor in order to bring it to normal pressure again, and then enter another device linked in series. I have not indicated all of the interconnections that might be used in such a system, but suffice it to say that if we have about a ten-stage system, it is possible to get 97 percent pure CO_2 delivered to space, or to any place you want to deliver it.

This system requires a considerable amount of power. It also requires considerable development in the state of the art in the preparation of membranes. The effective area of membrane required may be in the cate-

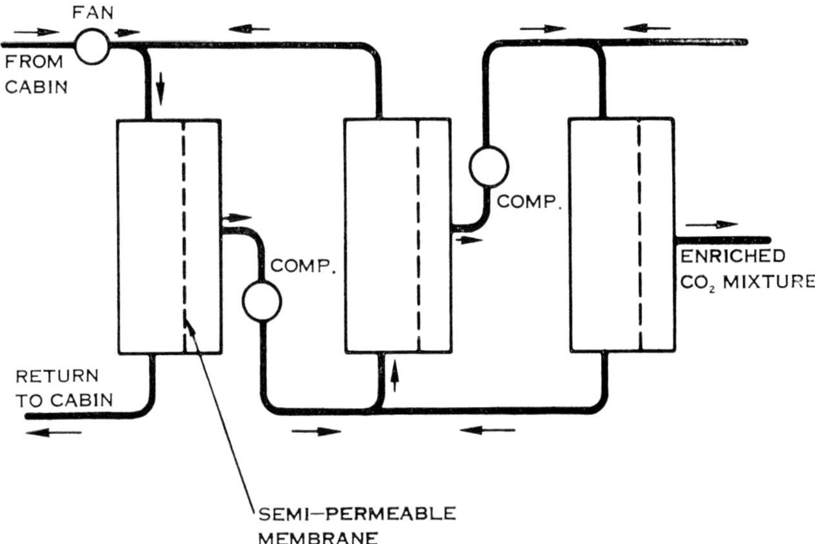

FIGURE 25. Semipermeable membrane concept for CO_2 separation.

gory of many thousands of square feet—it's not simply a matter of having a square foot of something like paper through which all of the CO_2 goes. It takes something more like a football field, well packaged into a small device.

Some important work has been reported recently on the development of membrane packages for multistage systems by Professor Major,[101] of the University of Akron, who has made some rather attractive epoxy-potted sandwiches of membranes, but which would still be subject to the disadvantage that the power required by the interstage compressors is rather sizable.

Ion exchange resins refer to a system in which the CO_2 laden cabin air passes through a bed of resins in which the CO_2 is absorbed, and then electrolytically transferred to another part of a liquid-containing cell (see FIGURE 26). We must have an ion exchange resin which can replace hydroxyl ions with carbonate ions (which can thereby absorb CO_2 through the release of water) and compress the potential between the two sides by making it part of a continuous cell. If this is an anion-permeable membrane, CO_2 can be absorbed, formed into a carbonate on the surface of the ion exchange resin, and pass through a second membrane

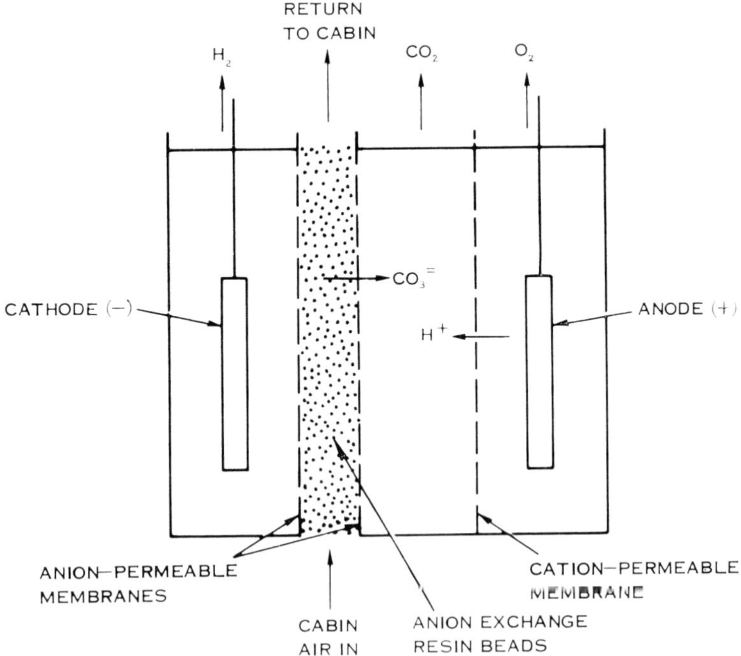

FIGURE 26. Ion exchange resin concept for CO_2 separation.

into a region which is separated from the final electrodes by a cation membrane. The cation-permeable membrane will permit hydrogen ions to pass in the other direction, and increase the acidity of this region of the cell, so that CO_2 will be released. It is necessary periodically to reverse the polarity in order to restore the capacity of the primary ion exchange resin for CO_2 absorption.

This system has been demonstrated, but to my knowledge has not been reduced to a practical operating system in terms of meeting space vehicle requirements, including zero gravity.

So far I have outlined the—let us call it the kindergarten level of CO_2 control in space vehicles in Phase II. It is necessary, though, to separate the concept of dumping CO_2 overboard, from dumping carbon overboard, from doing something that does not involve dumping carbon overboard.

In Phase III, we might use various chemical methods for oxygen reclamation from CO_2. There are four contenders for the honors of a chemically regenerable system in Phase III. The four are the Sabatier process, the Bosch process, the fused lithium carbonate electrolysis system, and the solid electrolyte system (see FIGURE 23).

The Sabatier process begins with the reaction of CO_2 and hydrogen to form methane and water. This is feasible as a one-step reaction, where water can be condensed out of the recirculating system and electrolyzed to produce hydrogen and oxygen. The oxygen, of course, is our desired product. The hydrogen produced can be returned for continued reaction with CO_2, except that the decomposition of water yields only two volumes of hydrogen, where we needed four volumes of hydrogen in the first place. Obviously we are throwing away methane, which contains hydrogen, and we have a deficiency to make up. So this is not the most attractive of regenerative systems, because we have a considerable requirement for the expenditure of a stored material, hydrogen.

However, the loss compared to the amount of oxygen recovered is 16 g. of material for 32 g. of oxygen, so it is a little bit better than throwing away all the CO_2

JENKINS: That system could be combined with a methane-fixing, bacterial system. This has been proposed, but no work has actually been done with it.

ARNOLDI: Actually, if you choose to decompose the methane as a second step in this system, then you have the Bosch system, which simply involves writing the equation: $CO_2 + 2H_2 \rightarrow C + 2H_2O$. This becomes an equilibrium reaction in which we can decrease the concentration of the reactants only slowly by removing the products. It involves the use of a catalyst in order to have a controllable reaction with a fairly decent yield.

It has a lot of characteristics that are similar to the Sabatier process, but it turns out to be fundamentally more complex to control, and therefore requires a higher level of engineering effort, of scientific effort, to develop it as a working system.

Work is going on currently on both of these systems. The preference seems to be for the Bosch process, although this is a matter of opinion among various investigators. A working system has been built and delivered to NASA at Langley for use in a space cabin simulator. By hearsay, I understand that the process is not all that is desired at the present time; that more work is necessary in order to bring it to the point where it could be qualified for space flights.

FENN: What temperatures are required for those two processes?

ARNOLDI: In the vicinity of 600°C.

FREMONT-SMITH: Could that Bosch system be driven in the direction you wanted to by heating one side of the reaction—having a temperature gradient across the reaction?

ARNOLDI: Yes. That turns out to be one of the important characteristics of the reactor here, that a temperature gradient is required, or at least in one concept a temperature gradient is required. This again complicates the process.

The process is also complicated by the fact that you have to remove the catalyst periodically and clean off the carbon deposited, and this is easy in concept but difficult in practice. In general, processes which involve collecting carbon on a catalyst involve permeation of carbon to the extent that the catalyst has to be regarded as an expendable, so the problem is to achieve a high ratio of carbon collected to the amount of catalyst present.

The third system, fused lithium carbonate electrolysis, is the one with which I am most familiar (see FIGURE 27).[102] Let me first describe it as being a system in which an electrolytic cell containing a fused mixture of alkali carbonates and alkali halides is electrolyzed so that the decomposed carbonates go to carbon at the cathode, oxygen at the anode, and an increased oxide ion concentration near the cathode. This increased oxide ion concentration makes it possible for the cell to absorb more CO_2 and thereby this becomes a one-step process which permits the CO_2 absorption directly from a cabin atmosphere CO_2 concentration, with the direct formation of the products in the cell.

This is unique in the sense that both the Sabatier and Bosch processes require previous concentration of the CO_2. They require the virtual elimination of oxygen from the gas to be processed in these techniques, and the preconcentration of CO_2 represents a considerable weight and power penalty.

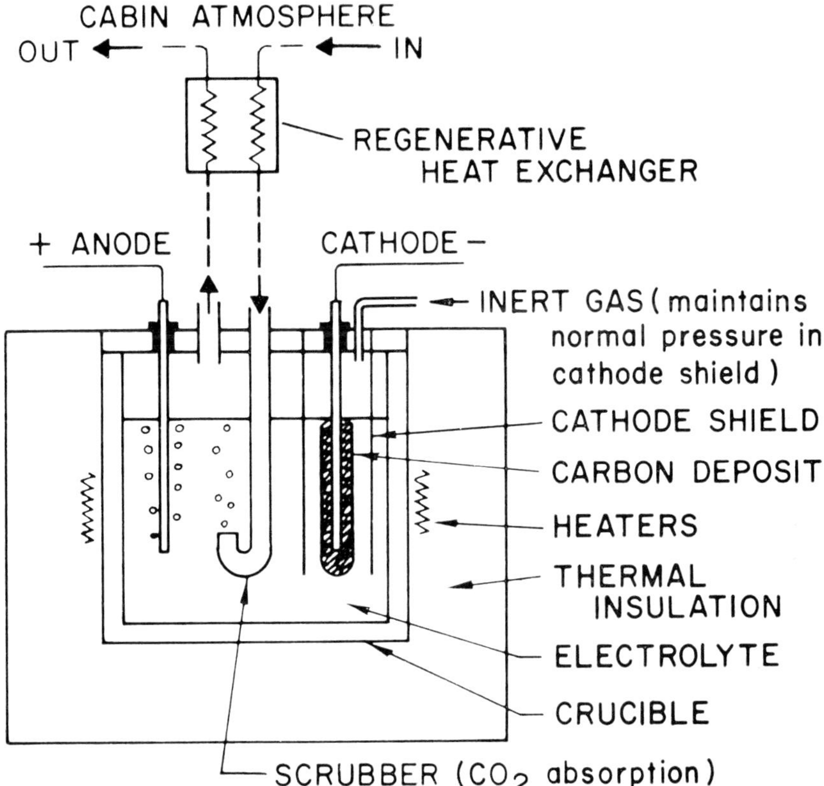

FIGURE 27. Schematic diagram CO_2 electrolytic cell.[102]

Let me describe the lithium carbonate process by writing a symbolic equation for the process (see FIGURE 23). Lithium carbonate yields lithium oxide plus carbon and oxygen. That does represent the overall process, together with the absorption of CO_2 to form lithium carbonate. The process is also attractive on the basis of a low power requirement.

The solid electrolyte system involves thermal decomposition of CO_2 to CO plus atomic oxygen plus the variety of miscellaneous compounds that you will get at about 1200°C. The solid electrolyte serves to separate the oxygen from this mixture and to deliver it in a useful form.

In a schematic sense, consider that we have a solid wall made of a polycrystalline mixture of certain oxides—commonly zirconium oxide and calcium oxide mixtures have been used, with a precious-metal electrode surface on each side of this wall (see FIGURE 28). Let us consider this to be a box into which we pass CO_2 and where the population of the molecules now includes CO_2, CO, and oxygen. At the interface, at tem-

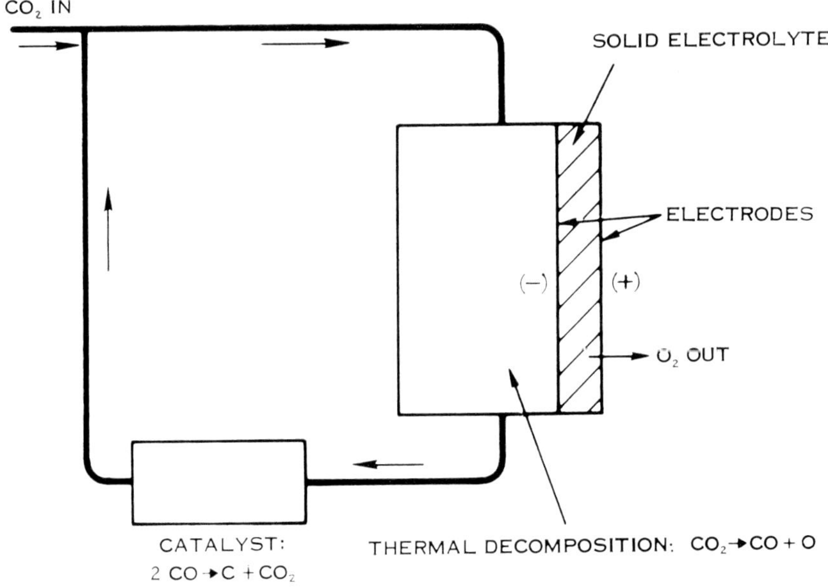

FIGURE 28. Solid electrolyte concept for CO_2 decomposition.

peratures like 1000 or 1200°C, oxygen will become ionized, will enter into vacancies in the crystal lattice structure, will be transported ionically from the negative to the positive electrode, and will be discharged as oxygen gas at the final electrode. This is quite analogous to what is referred to in aqueous chemistry as a concentration cell, only it happens to have a solid electrolyte, it is hot, and the entry of oxygen into the system comes from the initial thermal decomposition of CO_2.

The gases in the chamber need to be recirculated through a catalyst in which the disproportionation reaction takes place, whereby we can collect solid carbon and periodically dispose of it, with a certain amount of entrained catalyst. This gas, then, which is enriched in CO_2 needs to be circulated back through the entry to the thermal decomposition chamber. FIGURE 28 bears no resemblance at all to the physical embodiment of this concept. The physical embodiment generally involves a multiplicity of tubes with a solid electrolyte and gases are passed down the center of these tubes, and the oxygen emerges on the outside.

One of the difficulties in developing the system is not only the requirement for a high temperature, which makes for material stability problems and durability problems, but also the fact that two different temperatures are required in the system. We are recirculating gas from a 1200°C temperature in the decomposition chamber to a 600°C temperature in the catalyst. That means that for the sake of energy conservation, we have to add regenerative heat exchangers between the intake and the output of the catalyst bed, which adds to the equipment problems. It means also that we have to have a recirculating fan which works at a red-hot temperature, or near that, which is awkward—particularly bearings and seal problems, and so forth.

Nevertheless, this is a possible contender. There is CO involved in the system. However, the CO, at least as the system should operate, should never come in contact with the cabin gas. It should not be able to escape. If you put a crack through the electrolyte, of course, then you would have a problem, but I think in any of these systems you can postulate accidents which would be catastrophic.

I am not trying to express any preference for any one system. Of course, I like our own system better, but I can recognize that it has comparable disadvantages, or difficulties.

On the subject of temperature, let me point out that most of these are 600°C temperature systems, and this last one involves a temperature of around 1200°C. Some people like to talk about the possibility of going down in temperature, but the ionic conductivity of solid electrolytes falls off very rapidly, if you go very much below 1200°C, and it is unlikely that you can get very far down. From a strictly technical point of view you can get measurable conductivity as low as 600°C, but you cannot get much oxygen ion transport.

The fused carbonate system we have been running at temperatures in the vicinity of 550°C. This is mainly because we have not been able to figure out a good electrolytic mixture which would satisfy electrochemical requirements in the cell and at the same time have a low melting point. Theoretically the process could be run at a much lower temperature—even at room temperature—but we have not yet been able to devise a suitable solvent for the carbonate which will permit full ionization and which will permit control of certain decomposition pressures in the melt at room temperature. We have been able to operate such a system at temperatures as low as 375°C so far, but with serious compromises to the internal cell process.

I have been describing all of these systems in terms of a discrete unit operation. This does not necessarily represent the way it would be done with a multiple-man crew. Certainly in our electrolytic cell—just to make it sound foolish, let us consider that if you have a one-man oxygen reclamation system based on this process, and you accomplish the process in a single cell, the current requirement would be 100 amperes and the voltage would be in the vicinity of 2 volts. A 2-volt power supply that would deliver 100 amperes with suitable bus bars does not sound very good for a space vehicle. It is more likely that DC power would be available at 30 volts—maybe higher—and therefore a multiplicity of cells should be used, at least in theory, to match up with the components of the power supply.

There will probably be an optimum size of unit cell, an optimum module size, so that you will run a series parallel arrangement. This becomes like a collection of storage batteries hooked up in series and parallel, so as to achieve an optimum performance for a given type of duty.

The same thing holds true for a solid electrolyte cell. There is a necessity for an electrolyte which might be in tubular form; there would be a multiplicity of tubes, and there would certainly be some optimum modular element which would be cascaded into a system that would provide adequate capacity for whatever size of crew and type of mission we would have.

The Bosch and Sabatier processes, I believe, although I am not at all sure of this, would probably involve a similar breakdown into a modular concept.

Chemical Synthesis of Food

MAYER: I was surprised at the last conference [1] that I attended in Tampa, and again now, that it looks as though the only alternatives that are really contemplated in terms of nutrition are: either you take your food, or you produce it. But we do have a very large proportion of the world that is subsisting on a diet which has a very high proportion of carbohydrates, and certainly in rats you can maintain animals quite happily—adult rats—on, let us say, 85 percent of their diet coming from carbohydrates, 10 percent protein, and two or three percent fat.

Now, why is it not an alternative to either storing food or regenerating it, to take something like the Sabatier process, which gives you methane, which is a start in terms of chemical synthesis, and regenerate carbohydrate or conceivably simple molecules of butanediol, or something of that sort, which may have essentially the same nutritional value, and then do that chemically rather than biologically, which I think involves a great many more unknowns?

Then all you have to take along is some protein and some polyunsaturated fat, and maybe you regenerate your minerals. It seems to me you are saving 85 percent of your food space, and obviously there will be some machinery involved in terms of transforming methane into a usable, simple carbohydrate, but this is not an impossible problem.

ARNOLDI: I think your concept is probably valid. It becomes a matter of determining whether, with a finite expenditure of funds, such a system can be brought to a useful and reliable level of operation in time for a foreseeable mission.

MAYER: But it is being done. All the steps are known.

K. SCHWARZ: You mean to go chemically, catalytically, from methane to carbohydrate? That is one of the most difficult things to do, in good yield.

CALLOWAY: There is such a system under study now for NASA, I understand, and the products that they find it easy to make are glycerol, ethanol and, perhaps, fructose. Are you game to go with a mixture of fructose and ethanol?

MAYER: I have done it for years.

CALLOWAY: No, seriously, how much of these compounds are you willing to put in the system? The synthetic process is not so bad, if you can stop with glycerol or ethanol, but if you have to build larger molecules, there are multiple problems—yield, racemic mixtures, etc.

ARNOLDI: I have been carrying us through Phase III, or III½, or something around there, to get the chemical systems in perspective and in their place in the order of things. There is one generality that I would like to add to what I have remarked so far, which applies to all systems: It is inescapable, no matter what system you use, that to decompose CO_2 requires energy. There is a free energy change corresponding to the free energy of formation of CO_2 which is 94.4 kilocalories per gram mole, which is essentially independent of temperature.

This corresponds, for a man on a 3000-kilocalorie diet, to 100 watts of power. It takes about 100 watts per man, in other words, to decompose CO_2 to get the oxygen, and that is only 85 percent of the oxygen that he took in in the first place anyway.

JENKINS: Could you summarize what is the present status of these four processes with regard to present capability, or when it is anticipated that they might be available?

ARNOLDI: Well, present capabilities are represented by the fact that the Bosch process has been installed as hardware in the space capsule simulator at Langley. However, it has been having technical difficulties, and I would hesitate to say that it is a well-qualified system at this point.

The fused carbonate system is at a point in the process where we think we understand the principles involved, where we have solved a number of the problems, but where engineering development and design of a prototype system is still a bit in the future. We have working laboratory equipment which does produce carbon and oxygen, but our problem is to achieve sufficient understanding to exercise continuous control and assure reliability.

The solid electrolyte system, is, I believe, at a similar state, in the sense that working models have been made, but it is not yet a well-qualified prototype system.

The Sabatier process is really in a different category from the others. It really should not be compared with the others, because the product, methane, is a little bit different. It should be the most feasible of the processes, where it is eligible, but I do not know what the development status is.

MAYER: Would it be possible to make something which might be a better starting point for organic synthesis, to make acetylene instead of methane?

ARNOLDI: It certainly would be possible.

MAYER: It would take more current, but if you have a nuclear reactor as a source of power—

ARNOLDI: Well, you will get back what you pay for. And the state of the art in the various fields will determine what efficiencies you can achieve, so I would not say that you should be at all pessimistic on account of power. If you are going to produce food, you have to put energy in somehow.

However, as soon as you go into food production, the process becomes sufficiently more complicated that most engineers are inclined to shy off. In fact, they are inclined to find that the possibility of payoff in a finite time in the future is low enough that they cannot convince their management that it should be undertaken, much less NASA.

BROBECK: This may be because you are defining food too generally. If you defined food in a more limited way, the way Dr. Mayer has, it might work out very simply.

MAYER: There are some very simple molecules that might eventually replace carbohydrate as a source of up to 90 percent of the energy that is required. It seems to me that the thinking about food, except in the context that you just mentioned, has been very uncritical and not analytical enough. In adults ninety percent of the food is used essentially as a source of energy, and there is only 10 percent that has to be fairly specifically certain things.

ARNOLDI: I might make one peripheral comment on the subject of food production in the space vehicle. One of the criteria that has been applied to comparisons of systems has been based on the need to withstand a zero G environment, and that is a black mark against a system which involves liquids as well as gases and solids, and gives a considerable impetus to a solid electrolyte system involving only the solid and gaseous phase, or the Bosch system.

A number of chemical processes which might produce the elements of a food supply—in the sense that you are saying now—may involve the use of aqueous solutions. Process control is difficult in subsystem parts where there needs to be an interface between a liquid solution and a gas —certainly an all-gas system would be much more attractive for zero gravity requirements.

I think the requirement for zero gravity operation is often being overemphasized, and people are overpessimistic about the use of liquid-gas interfaces in a zero gravity situation, but, nevertheless, it is a fact of life that it is difficult to sell—to convince somebody against his will that a liquid-containing system does not have serious disadvantages.

MAYER: Well, of course, the minute you start thinking of synthesis of amino acids, you are involved in all sorts of liquid–gas problems, but as long as you limit it to carbon, hydrogen, and oxygen, it may be relatively simple.

Bioregenerative Systems

JENKINS: On a molecular weight basis these processes would waste about half a pound of carbon per person per day. This is to be eliminated either as methane or as elemental carbon or as carbon lost in a sieve or filter. They also involve fairly high temperatures—550 up to 1200 °C—and there are some poisonous gases involved. Nevertheless, they are further ahead than the bioregenerative systems. They do not presently involve food; but, as Dr. Mayer has pointed out, some of the materials could be utilized in the formation of food.

Bioregenerative systems operate at low temperatures. Both the bacterial and the photosynthetic systems operate at room temperature, and there are no toxic, poisonous materials involved, other than the potential toxic materials which might be involved in the plants themselves, or the bacteria. Here we have a system which takes up the carbon dioxide, gives off oxygen, and can produce food and can utilize at least a part of the wastes, particularly the urine. I do not think anyone is thinking in terms of supplying 100 percent of the food requirement, but there is a possibility that some of the products might be used as part of the food requirement.

POLLARD: How long does it take to get a bioregenerative system up to full activity?

My reason for asking this is: what if it should go toxic and become unreactive? Could you take lyophilized starter colonies and start a new system? How long does it generally take to get up to a point where you are producing the required number of grams per millimeter?

JENKINS: In the case of bacteria, the production time for a new generation is about three to four hours, and there is a small lag phase in this system.

Dr. Ward, what is this for algae?

WARD: It depends on the environmental conditions. If you had to start a new culture of a thermotolerant strain you could get a doubling rate of eight or nine at light saturation. At eight or nine doublings per day of your population, it would not take very long—I would say, 24 hours or so —to reach a population that would be functional again.

D. SCHWARZ: I think that in this situation you might very well, just as insurance, have a standard procedure for running a seed stock pretty steadily, which would be tantamount to reculturing your stock culture at regular intervals, just to protect from this. That would not be much of a weight penalty or a great problem.

JENKINS: In other words, have a complete harvest, clean out, and actually go into a batch stage.

D. SCHWARZ: Always have a partially developed seed stock, just to protect yourself against this and cut down on delay time.

POLLARD: Of course, even there you might be getting into a mutational drift.

JENKINS: And this would be the value of having seed stock.

BROBECK: Can this not be done in units, like batteries, so that a change that affects one is not going to affect all of them?

WARD: That is a popular concept. The system could be run in separate units rather than as a completely mixed culture.

BROWN: I think algal and bacterial systems are not really different here, in the sense that the time to get up to speed is relatively short—measured in hours, not days. Probably fixing whatever went wrong would take more time than getting the system going again, and you would almost necessarily have duplicate units.

D. SCHWARZ: I think the basic principle of redundancy has to be built into this system, whatever you use. It is inconceivable to make any kind of a system work that has no redundancy, or no balance in it.

JENKINS: I can see a system using both bacteria and algae.

I would like to call on Dr. Ward now for a very brief discussion of the algal system.

WARD: I would like to preface my remarks by saying that my colleague, Dr. Richard L. Miller, and I have reviewed elsewhere most of the material to be presented.[103]

The subject of bioregeneration apparently originated in 1951 when Dr. Heinz Specht, at an Air Force symposium on the physics and medicine of the upper atmosphere, suggested that man's respiratory requirements might be supplied by photosynthesis of green plants. Following this initial suggestion, several plant physiologists, primarily Dr. Jack Myers at the University of Texas, attempted to calculate reasonable estimates of the logistics of the process. Numerous demonstration-type experiments followed which amounted to qualitative repetitions of the Priestley experiment. In other words, the respiratory requirements of a mouse were more or less supplied by an actively growing culture of algae.

At present I view the field of photosynthetic regeneration as having gone through three fairly distinct phases of development. We are currently in the third phase.

Stage one consisted of the early logistics calculations, selection of algae as the plants best suited for regenerative purposes, and demonstration experiments using simple apparatus readily put together in the laboratory. Work during this phase was done almost entirely by biologists over a period of three to four years with very low research budgets. In contrast, stage two mostly involved the efforts of engineers in various companies, lasted about eight years, and consumed large amounts of government research funds. The engineering community felt, and justifiably so, that they could offer significant improvement over the relatively unsophisticated efforts of the biologists on, what to a large extent is, a chemical engineering problem. The engineers produced many manuscripts, most of them buried in company reports and files, and arrived at, what I consider to be, a very unsatisfactory state of the art. They made a number of excellent contributions, but in general failed to appreciate the biology of the organisms with which they were dealing. Following stage two, government support for photosynthetic regeneration research was drastically reduced. Now I believe we are in stage three, where we recognize that it is going to require the efforts of both biologists and engineers working together to define the parameters needed for successful development. Although current research on algal systems is now limited to only a few laboratories, I feel that progress is being made toward realistic development and evaluation.

Numerous algal systems have been designed and tested during the last 10 or so years. Culture containers have included panels, cylinders, tanks, and many others. One of the first tasks was to define adequately the factors that limit algal growth in mass culture, such as temperature, carbon dioxide, and mineral nutrients. Once adequate specifications for these factors were determined, it became apparent that development of algal regenerative systems is largely a problem in illumination engineering. Artificial light sources have received the greatest attention, supposedly, because of the engineering difficulties of using sunlight in space.

JENKINS: At least in a spacecraft.

WARD: Yes, in a spacecraft. A lunar colony would be another matter. However, appropriate locations on the moon are limited. Even in a location with a 12-hour light-dark cycle the design parameters for an algal system would automatically be double.

The fluorescent lamp, with an efficiency of about 20 percent, is the most efficient commercially available light source. The maximum efficiency of a green plant system in converting light energy into chemical energy is about 20 percent. A 20 percent efficiency can only be demonstrated under carefully controlled conditions that permit light of low intensity to be completely absorbed. These conditions would not operate in a gas exchanger of practical size. Hence, the *maximum* theoretical electrical efficiency would be $0.2 \times 0.2 = 0.04$ or 4 percent. The rest of the energy goes into heat. It is evident that photosynthetic systems are severely limited with respect to efficiency, especially so, since practical efficiencies seldom exceed half the theoretical maximum.

The primary advantage of the algal system is plasticity of design. It is possible to decrease size by increasing power input; however, if you want efficiency the size becomes larger. These relationships can be seen in FIGURE 29. Dr. Miller and I tried to convert the experimental data available in the literature to common units of expression, such as grams dry algae produced per unit energy, area and volume. We used a simplified

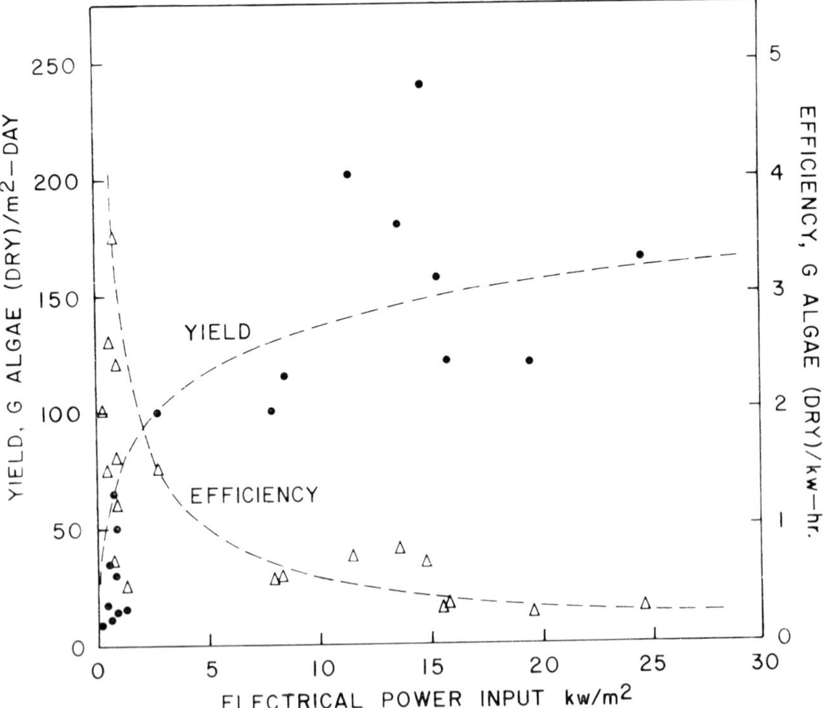

FIGURE 29. Yield per unit area and efficiency as a function of electrical power input for illumination.[103]

form of the Bush equation to calculate the theoretical curves and resorted to what one might call qualitative mathematics. Data given are actual experimental results that have been published in the literature. So we have grams dry algae/m^2-day and efficiency in terms of dry algae/kW-hr plotted against electrical power input in kW/m^2.

JENKINS: The meter square is illumination surface?

WARD: Yes, the surface area of the culture exposed to light.

It is obvious that there is an inverse relationship between efficiency and energy input. The most efficient systems require a large culture volume exposed to low intensity light over a large surface area. It is possible to obtain extremely high yields per unit surface or volume by increasing energy input; however, you sacrifice electrical efficiency which, as Mr. Arnoldi previously indicated, can be converted to weight at a projected value of 20 lb. per kilowatt. I believe that we can now make an approximately accurate estimate of the power requirements of an algal system. Weight requirements are another thing entirely. I personally place little confidence in any of the weight comparisons of various systems simply because I do not know of one system that has been built for that purpose. Most systems have not been designed for efficiency either.

There have been few regenerative systems built for reliability in the laboratory and none for projected reliability in a space mission. However, several algal systems have performed reliably for periods of months in the laboratory—Dr. Krauss has an excellent example—and have been managed for steady-state output. I do not know of a chemical system that has been demonstrated to be reliable for a period of months. On paper they look good. As far as demonstrations of reliability go, I believe that the algal system is probably more advanced than any chemical system.

FIGURE 30 represents the approximate "state of the art" in the development of algal systems. Curves were again calculated from the Bush equation and represent light sources of 10 and 20 percent efficiency. Surface area values are those required to produce 600 g. dry algae per day. It can be shown that one liter of oxygen is liberated for each gram of algae produced. Therefore, using a reasonable value of 600 liters of oxygen per man per day, an algal system must be capable of producing 600 grams of algae per day. We can see then, that surface area can be reduced significantly by increasing power input, but only with a tremendous sacrifice in efficiency.

Provided adequate space for culture apparatus is available, a power requirement of about 10 kW per man would be reasonable. Using Mr. Arnoldi's figure of 20 lb. per kW we obtain a value of 200 lb. as the weight of the power system to support one man.

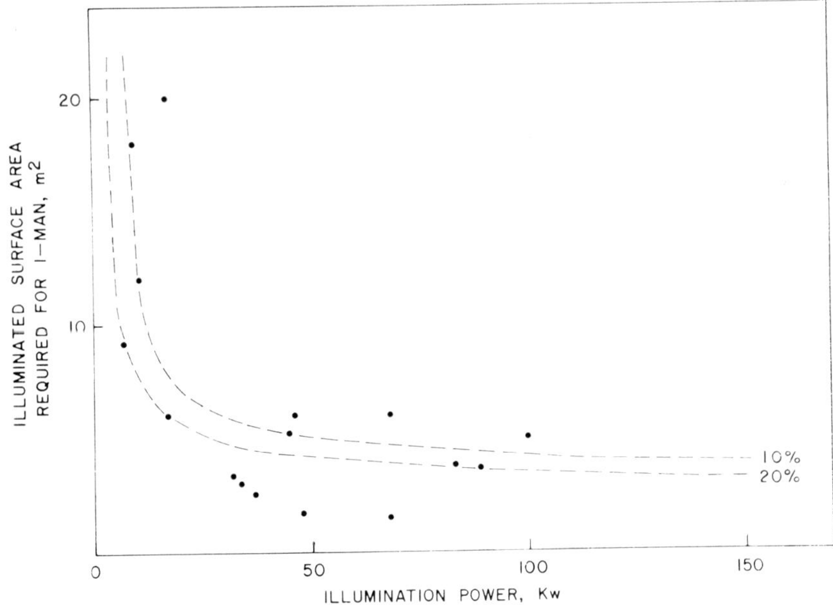

FIGURE 30. Illuminated surface area required for one-man support as a function of illumination power.[103]

Because of low efficiency and the fact that the engineering community is basically skeptical of any biological system for regeneration, the algal system is no longer considered by many to be a serious contender for space application. In fact, photosynthetic regeneration was recently referred to as a "technologic will-o-the-wisp" in a leading aerospace engineering technical magazine. However, in summary I would like to quote Dr. Edward Teller from his lecture at the NASA Conference in Tampa, Florida. He said:

> "Nuclear energy provides a very ample supply of energy, and it is entirely permissible—particularly in a fixed base—to use this energy wastefully. In fact, practically the only problem is how to get rid of the energy, or to cool it, once it is created; therefore, when designing the intricate, important, and hopefully, light units for food synthesis, I think it would be well if it is assumed that as much energy as desired can be obtained. Don't economize on energy. Economize on weight."

He further indicated that before we undertake a long-duration mission such that regeneration would be required, that we will have to provide energy in such large quantities for other functions that energy expended for life support would be somewhat incidental.

There will undoubtedly be many engineering reasons for selection of one life support system over another. I believe the primary criterion will be reliability rather than efficiency or weight.

BROWN: The thinking has changed as the booster capability has increased, and just as we are talking now about several men going to the moon, whereas only a few years ago we were talking about trying desperately to get one grapefruit into orbit—if we compare the payloads that have been used in the past and those that are just on the horizon, the difference is very large. If I remember the numbers, the Mercury capsule was something like 2500 lb., and the payload for Saturn V in earth orbit is something of the order of 30 or 40 tons. So payloads have gone up, and they probably, if we extrapolate 20 years, will go up further.

Now, this is from one standpoint a reason to forget about regeneration. We know that we can feed people on stored food and water, stored oxygen, CO_2 absorbents. If we have the payload capacity, let us do it.

This is not necessarily the best solution from the engineering standpoint, let alone the biological standpoint, because the payload space is never going to be free. You are always going to have some competition, and I am personally convinced that other factors than weight are sure to be determining when the decisions are finally made, if they are made on a logical basis.

Also, there is a lot of folklore about algalburgers not being fit to eat, and there have been a few unpleasant experiences of people who have tried to eat algae, and other things, and have gotten sick on it; and if you talk to anyone, particularly an engineer who has not had much elbow-rubbing with biologists, they are afraid of the fact that biology is mysterious and maybe the algae will die. They are much more confident in predicting lifetimes of catalysts than they are of biological systems. If you talk to a biochemical engineer, he has a somewhat different attitude.

Now, if we think of the magnitude of the job to be done in terms of the weight that you have to invest, the biggest job, of course, is water, and everyone accepts the fact that it will be recycled. We are not going to carry fresh water for a Martian mission.

If we are concerned only with the gas exchange, the oxygen–CO_2 management and nothing else for the moment, and if we can solve that problem, then we have solved most of our weight problems.

So you could forget about all of the nutritional aspects and the same arguments would go on between the bacterial and the algal and the various chemical systems. They would go on in almost the same way as they have been going on.

I think there are three criteria that ought to be a basis for making a decision ultimately. We do not have the information on any of these criteria to make a decision now.

First would be the adequacy of the system to meet steady-state requirements. In terms of the paper chemistry and the arithmetic involved, there are no doubts that any one of these systems can do the job, or most of the job.

The second point is one of reliability, and we are never going to know the answer to this until you have test models that you can subject to long-term tests.

The third criterion is going to be weight, and I am equating power to weight here. They are not quite interchangeable, but for our purposes I think we can assume that they are.

And if you put all three together, no one of them is going to determine the solution. It may turn out that an algal system is slightly lighter—or a lot lighter—than, let us say, a bacterial system; and yet for quite different reasons you may decide to use the bacterial system. But weight is going to be a factor in the decision all the way up to the time when we are actually on our way to Mars with it.

Well, I think we could spend a lot of time going over ground that has been plowed over and over again on the engineering details, and we would not be talking nutrition, and that is what most of the group here, I think, would prefer to talk about. I think we need a very general background, and Mr. Arnoldi certainly gave us this on the chemical systems. This from what I know, is a very good summary. We know in general what is possible. We know in general what the limitations are; but we do not—and will not until the state of the art has progressed somewhat—know exactly what, for example, the number of pounds per man would be for these different systems. But we now have ballpark figures, and all of them are in the running.

However, if we think of systems as doing much more than just manage oxygen and carbon dioxide—think of them as producing part of the astronaut's diet—then I think we are getting closer to the area of competence and interest of most of the people here.

Well, when we do this I would like to emphasize that we are dealing not just with man as one of the components of the system, but man plus his flora. To my knowledge there have been very few attempts even to do nutritional studies on algae or bacteria of the sort that will have to be done. There have been very sporadic attempts, and I think it is significant that the main limitation here is the availability of algae—and I mean algae produced aseptically, so you are not eating Salmonella, yeast, and other things—or bacteria. This is something that I hope NASA is working on, but, frankly, I have not seen the evidence that this is a high-priority item. You are not going to move very fast in this direction until there are large quantities of dependable material to feed rats and other experimental animals, including man.

Now, we heard some discussions of the way man and his flora interact and some of the problems we can get into if that flora is disturbed. It seems most reasonable to expect his flora to be disturbed by a very drastic change in the diet, and we have no baseline information here at all, so there is a lot of work to be done of the kind that you do not ordinarily think about, on subjects which are living on, for example, bacteria as a major or complete dietary supplement.

Another uncertainty which I think we should pay some attention to is the possibility of using the algae or bacteria, or even Dr. Mayer's synthetic food as a beginning of a food chain which would include more animals than men. This has been proposed a number of times in the past. It has been rejected almost out of hand by people who do the simple calculation that your efficiency goes way down if you start introducing other components in the food chain. It has been thought very attractive—and, I think, for inadequate reasons—by those who say: Well, I refuse to eat algae, but I am willing to eat chickens, and if you will feed the algae to the chickens, this is fine—it will solve the problem.

I think both of these viewpoints are much too superficial, and I would not like to see the concept of a food chain consisting of more than just the one organism—man—dismissed without more investigation of it. There is no magic number for weight of the algal systems, but I bracket it in a range between two and ten times the weight of the man. What is your estimate, Dr. Ward?

WARD: I prefer a very conservative estimate of 1000 lb. per man. I think 500 lb. might be more realistic, but to be on the safe side I use 1000 lb. As I said before, I do not know of a system that has been designed with weight as a primary criterion. Our work has stressed reliability, regardless of weight. We are in the process now of completing a very elegantly designed algal system with the capability of supporting the respiratory requirements of two men continuously. The system should be in operation within a few months and will be used for actual life support experiments—not for food supply in the beginning, nor will we attempt to recycle mineral nutrients or achieve a chemical balance, but for atmosphere control and demonstration of long duration reliability. This will be the first really hard engineering attempt that I know of to define the parameters governing the operation of a man-supportive algal system.

FENN: Would this system operate in zero G also?

WARD: The system as designed would not. However, the design principles used could easily be adapted to zero gravity operation.

FENN: It would take more weight still, though?

WARD: No, not unless there is a basic effect of weightlessness on algal metabolism which we cannot predict. In our system algal cells are suspended in a liquid medium. The culture is pumped through illumination panels. Liquid–gas contact—getting CO_2 to the algal cells—is accomplished with gravity independent methods. Liquid–gas separation—removal of oxygen from the liquid suspension—is accomplished in a centrifugal separator. The principles we are using could be adapted for operation in an environment free of gravity.

MUNRO: Is the figure of a thousand pounds the weight of the system per man? This could be compared with the per man, per year requirement for oxygen plus dried food of only about 500 kilograms.

WARD: Dr. Krauss will talk about the work done on the use of algae for animal and human food. He recently wrote an excellent review on the subject. I do not think we should hope to have man existing on a total algal diet, although it would be beneficial for chemical balance of the life support system.

KRAUSS: Regrettably, the time is very short. I think that a whole Conference could be devoted to some of the questions we are touching on this morning. There has been almost a subjective reaction in certain quarters with regard to bioregenerative systems. There appears to be a feeling that the by-product of the bioregenerative system, whether it is an alga or a bacterium, is going to be pretty unacceptable, and on that basis perhaps we had better move forward and give the examination of these things fairly low priority.

Rather than read into the record all of the data that we now have available with regard to the nutritive levels of algae, I have passed around this morning a reprint of a review of the field, which I wrote several years ago, which I think is essentially complete.[104] It discusses what we know about the nutritive value of the algae, and what very little indeed we know about the acceptability of this sort of food.

I might say, however, that the algae are fairly tractable and can be modified in culture or processed afterwards. I wish I had brought along a processed sample of these organisms which looks like flour essentially. It is white, odorless, tasteless, and about 70 percent protein. What the food technologists could do with material of this sort as a food source, of course, remains to be seen.

However, I do not feel that the major problem concerning the use of a product of a bioregenerative system is the problem of turning this material into something of value which is thoroughly acceptable for nutrition. The problems are the problems which Dr. Ward touched upon this morning,—the engineering of a system which is reliable and adequate and reasonably compressible into the limitations of the space capsule.

To give some estimate of what we are dealing with, I made a few calculations on the basis of some of Mr. Arnoldi's figures this morning, and also on the basis of some of the figures of Drs. Ward and Jenkins.

Dr. Jenkins pointed out that for a three-year mission for a crew of ten, the requirement would be a total of something in the neighborhood of 100,000 kilograms for life support.

Now, using Mr. Arnoldi's figure of energy available—something like 20 lb. of generating system per kilowatt of energy—and calculating in turn the amount of weight required for an algal system—knowing the production of that algal system and assuming that about 100 l. of culture plus supporting apparatus excluding an energy supply would be required per man—I have been able to come up with a figure which gives you at least an idea of why bioregeneration looks so attractive.

First of all, let me say that I have used a figure of 500 lb. of culture plus supporting material per man, instead of Dr. Ward's 1000 lb. Consequently, my figures are somewhat less conservative than his by 50 percent, but if one makes the appropriate calculations one comes up with something like a requirement of 4½ tons for a regenerating system including the energy source to supply the man for this period of flight, in contrast to 120 tons that he would have to carry along if he were indeed using stored supplies.

Even if you say: Well, Mr. Arnoldi's figure of 20 is a hopeful one—that perhaps 50 is better in terms of pounds per kilowatt—one still does not get too discouraging a figure. If the figure becomes 10 or 12 tons per man, you are still an order of magnitude better for a bioregenerative system. This is why bioregeneration is attractive and why some of us feel that it has been somewhat neglected.

When one comes to just what the bioregenerative system is, one deals rather quickly with some very severe problems. My own personal belief is that too much reliance on estimates of efficiency can lead one into rather dangerous conclusions. Basically, what we must look at is how efficient a system is in producing organic matter as reduced carbon—which, in a cell, can be considered equivalent to food. If we understand this completely and base our estimates on the reliability of this production, we are also able to come up with realistic estimates with regard to gas exchange.

Earlier, in the consideration of photosynthetic systems for life support, the emphasis tended to be on the amount of oxygen that could be produced by a given weight or a given volume of algae per hour. The algae can under certain circumstances produce a great deal more oxygen than they might be assumed to produce on the basis of the amount of carbon that they are reducing. In other words, for a while we thought that we could force the algae to spin their wheels, so to speak, to put out oxygen and we could be less concerned about their growth. However, it must be clear that you have got to do something with the hydrogen that is split from water. What you do with the hydrogen is reduce carbon. The product of this process is food of some sort—carbohydrate, fat, protein, and so forth. In the algal cell only a small part is undigestible polysaccharide. So I think we must concentrate on how much production of material one of these bio-regenerative systems may give.

In order to orient you about bioregeneration with algae, I would like to show you a couple of pictures to give you a very quick idea of what a bioregenerative system is, and then just a couple of illustrations which might show up some of our problems.

First of all just so you will know what these organisms look like, FIGURE 31 shows a group of fairly typical algal cells, and there are probably some thirty species of *Chlorella* which are potential candidates. This is an algal cell about 5 microns in diameter with a fairly large chloroplast, but with a good deal of the cell being devoted to cytoplasm. Now, with selection of species you can come up with organisms that have very large, massive parietal chloroplasts, and those which would

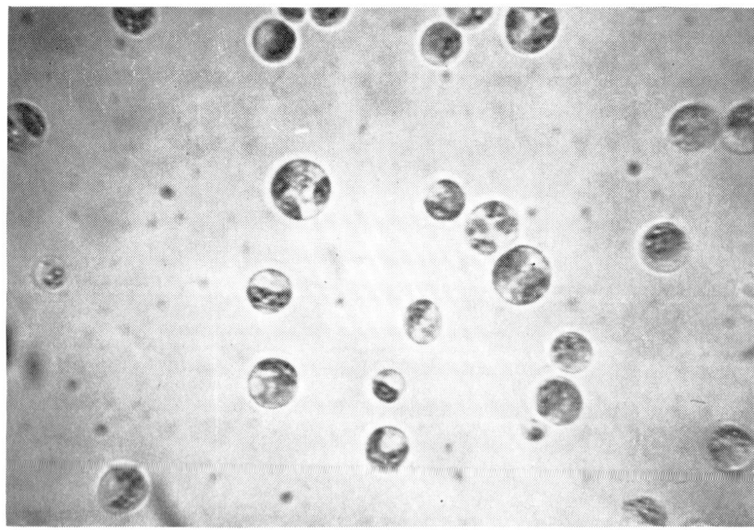

FIGURE 31. *Chorella candida* Shihiri and Krauss cultured on an inorganic medium in the light showing normal chloroplast and light-green pigmentation. × 900.

have very small ones. With the modification media you can change the chloroplast size, the carbohydrate/protein ratios, etc.

When the same organism is being handled in a different kind of medium, the chloroplast has essentially vanished, and one has a white organism now that can be readily utilized, and much of the taste and odor that comes from a green chlorophyl system is quite missing under these conditions.

Our lab has been concerned with basic problems. We have not tried to produce a photosynthetic gas exchanger, but for various purposes we have had to grow algae in large amounts, and this is to give you some idea of the instrumentation involved in producing algae. FIGURE 32 shows the device which we call the recyclostat, which is something like a chemostat, except that it recycles the water.

In other words, one does not just run medium through a standing culture. One conserves all of that medium and recycles it. I thought you might be interested in seeing some of the elements, because in the space vehicle we are going to have to go through some type of recycling system, and this may be somewhat like it. It can apply equally well to bacteria or algae.

Almost all of the data now in the literature which are concerned with the growth rates and yields of algae, have been collected from experiments with culture systems that do not involve the principle of recycling. Test tube cultures, in which the initial medium is gradually absorbed by the organism and in which the population expands to a given limit, are the most common culture vessels. The more sophisticated chemostat and photocell-monitored continuous-culture devices, although providing for a constant population, maintain that population by progressive dilution with fresh medium and discard of the old medium. Neither of these approaches is satisfactory for a space system where recycling of the water and the meduim is necessary. Consequently, the Recyclostat has been developed in our laboratory. The employment of this type of continuous culture system imposes rigorous demands on the performance of the culture, maintenance of sterility, and the nutrient replacement formula, but allows experiments to be done with the kind of conservative device which will be necessary for space. A brief description of the Recyclostat is given in FIGURE 33 and was included in NASA publication SP-70.[1]

Currently, studies are under way which are designed to answer the question of how growth rates and yields of cultures perform when light intensity and cell concentration are varied. It is important to know not only the maximum attainable yields—which will determine oxygen evolution—but, also, to know what yields can be expected if the organisms

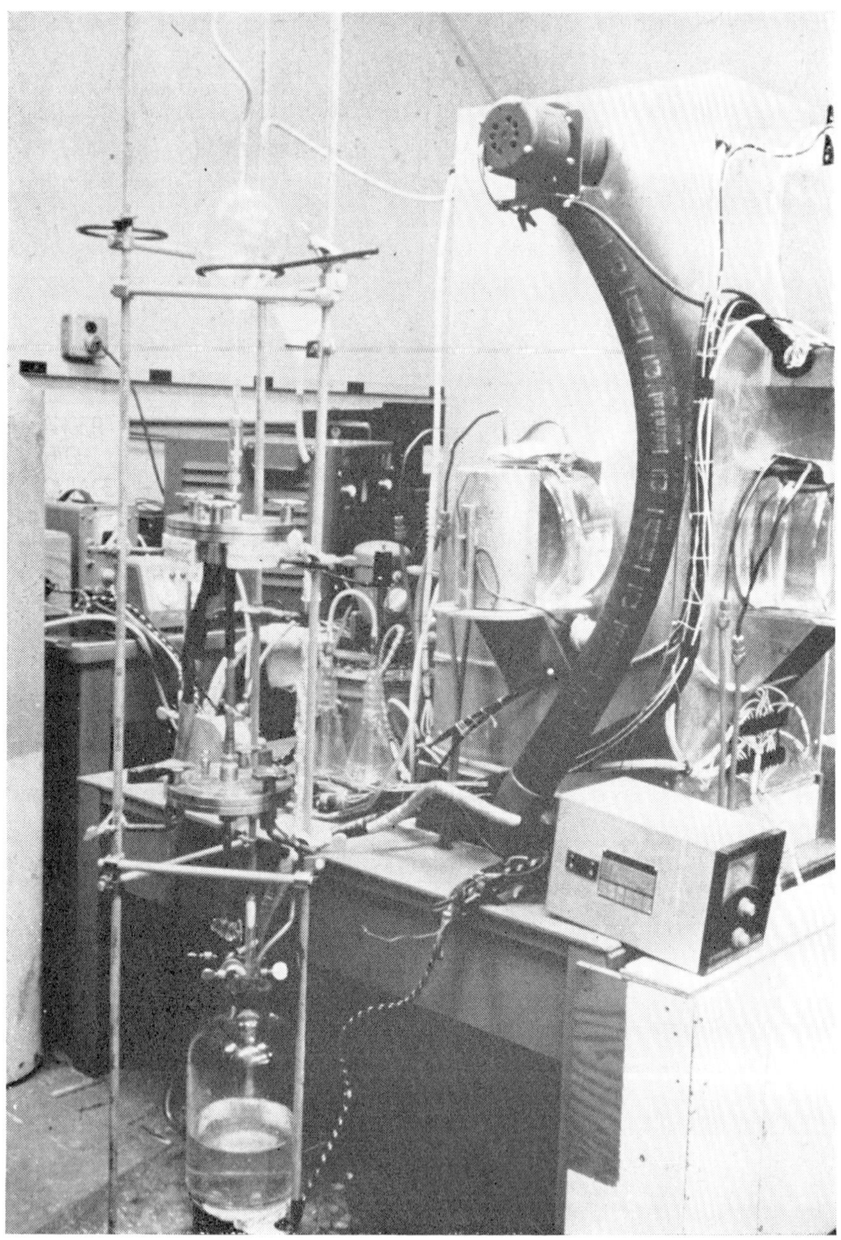

FIGURE 32. The Recyclostat: an automatically recycling, continuous sterile culture apparatus for algae and other microorganisms. Designed to provide data on the growth of organisms cultured for long periods of time in which the medium is replaced only with inorganic nutrients and all water is recycled.

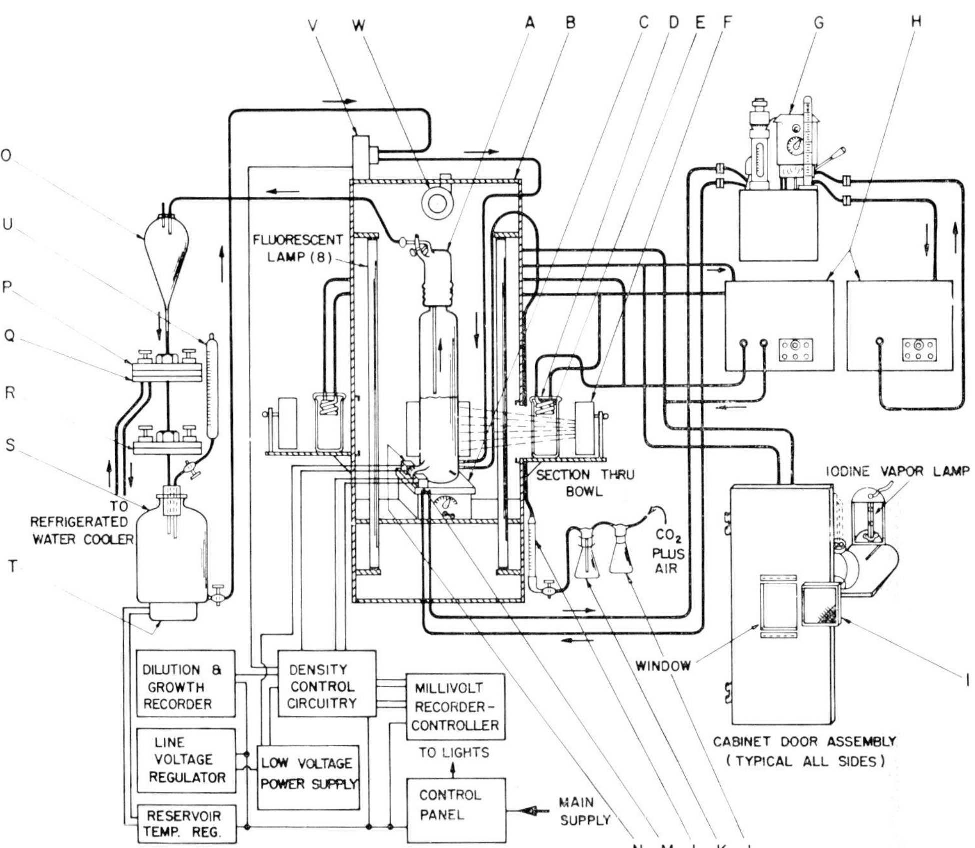

FIGURE 33. The Recyclostat: a continuous cultural apparatus for experiments on algae in sterile recycled media under controlled light and temperatures. The system provides for sterile culture, harvest, and recycling of medium which is continuous and automatic. A, culture chamber (including top and bottom as one callout); B, cabinet; C, electric stirrer; D, water filter; E, cooling coil; F, high-intensity "Quartzline" iodine vapor lamp; G, temperature regulator; H, potentiometer; J, water cooler; K, gas filter, cottom; L, gas filter, water; M, flow meter; N, photo duo diode; O, reference lamp (V_2); P, vacuum pump; Q, timer; R, stopcocks; S, recycled medium reservoir; T, solenoid (L_1); vacuum trap; V, intermediate supernatant reservoir; W, membrane bacterial filter; X, overflow receiver; Y, flow inductor; Z, fluorescent lamp.

must be maintained at suboptimal levels. The preparation of reliable long term data of this kind requires a major effort. The work with the low temperature *Chlorella vannielii* is nearing completion and the data at hand are summarized and plotted in FIGURE 34.

The data show an optimum optical density of near 1.0, a dry weight of 0.65 g./liter and a yield of 1.2 gram dry weight/liter/day. Data, which can be compared to test tube cultures at absolute maxima, show that

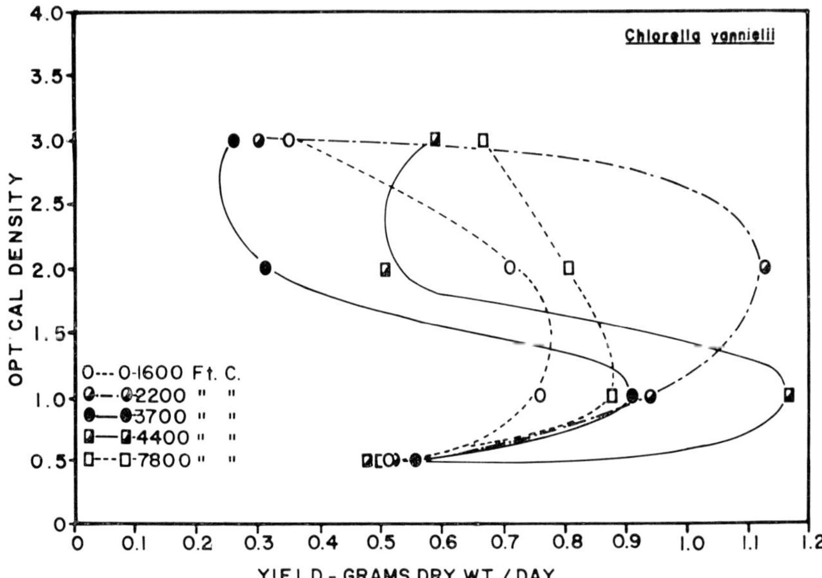

FIGURE 34. The yield of *Chlorella vannielii* related to optical density and light intensity in long-term Recyclostat experiments at 25°C. Cultures are bacteriafree and growth has been continually monitored and plotted on a recorder.

at this rate 436 liters of culture would suffice to supply the O_2 requirement of one man in a sealed chamber (see TABLE 19). In tubes with a larger surface area 290 liters would suffice.

Such data must be employed with an understanding of the basic growth equations which determine the optimum yields possible with a system of static population density—such as the one derived by Krauss and Osretkar in 1961.[105] They further show that increases in efficiency can be achieved by increasing the illuminated surface area. However, from an engineering point of view this may be undesirable. In our studies the design of the Recyclostat is such that the greatest possible number of variables can be examined. The utilization of all of the light energy has not been attempted. Consequently, a relatively small portion of the illumination available in the chamber is intercepted by the algal culture. Without correcting for the nonabsorbed light, the efficiency is 0.1 percent of the kilowatts employed.

Studies are also under way with the high-temperature strain *Chlorella sorokiniana*. The first long-term data are now available and demonstrate clearly the relation between cell concentration, growth rate, and yield at 1600 foot candles at 38°C. At this level no significant increase in yield is evident—the maximum still being at 1.2 g./liter/day (see

TABLE 19

COMPARISON OF RATES AND YIELDS OF *Chlorella vannielii* IN THE RECYCLOSTAT AND IN TEST TUBES AS RELATED TO HUMAN O_2 REQUIREMENTS

	Recyclostat Equivalents (8 cm. diameter)	Test-Tube Equivalents (2 cm. diameter)
Algal Growth Rate Doublings/Day	2.7	3.3
Optical Density	1.0	1.5
Maximum Algal Yield Grams Dry Wt./Liter/Day	1.0	1.5
O_2 Liters/Gram Algae	1.4	1.4
O_2 Requirement Liters/Man/Day	610.0	610.0
Algal Volume Required for O_2 One Man/Day	436.0	291.0
Surface Area—cm^2/Liter	440.0	1760.0
Algal Illuminated Surface Sq. Meters/Man/Day	19.3	51.2

FIGURE 35). It must be kept in mind that the data are now being compiled for constant turbulence and surface area. Equations will be developed for these factors once the baseline for light intensity/cell concentration is established. There is no doubt that the yield in terms of liters necessary per man, as well as the efficiency will be much more promising when the study is completed. When they are completed they will be the only accurate, long-term, sterile, recycled experiments in the literature.

Hydrogenomonas eutropha System

JENKINS: If there is time this afternoon, we might come back to this but I would like to take just a few minutes to review the bacterial system, involving *Hydrogenomonas eutropha.*

This system involves three things: the astronaut, the bacteria, and the electrolysis. This process is different from the photosynthetic process, in that instead of having about a 4 percent efficient system, we have an electrolysis system which is effective in cutting water into oxygen and hydrogen with about 80 percent efficiency. *Hydrogenomonas* uses some of the oxygen plus all of the hydrogen and carbon dioxide; the nutrient medium is urine supplemented with magnesium and ferrous iron.

This produces food which perhaps can be used by the astronauts,

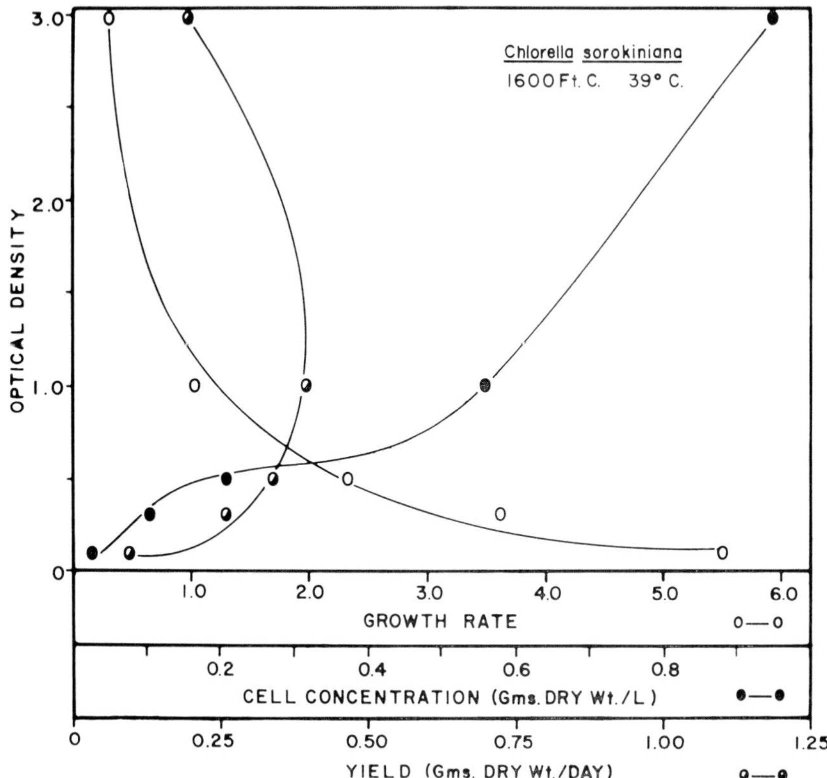

FIGURE 35. The yield of *Chlorella sorokiniana* related to optical density and growth rate in long-term Recyclostat experiments at 38°C. Cultures are bacteriafree and growth has been continually monitored and plotted on a recorder.

and pure oxygen. It requires about 20 l. per man at about 10 g. of dry bacteria per liter to support a man.*

These bacteria are composed of about 70–85 percent protein. However, if you grow these organisms in a medium which is deficient in either oxygen or nitrogen, you can produce cells that contain up to 80 percent of lipid, chiefly poly-beta-hydroxybutyric acid. If a lower protein food were desirable, a system could be devised in which a portion of the culture was managed in such a way as to yield more lipid. However, the nutritional properties of the lipid are not known.

I would like now to call on Dr. Calloway to tell us where we stand with regard to this problem of the bacteria as a potential for food.

* Additional information on culture conditions will be found in Volume I of this series. Ed.

K. SCHWARZ: Could I ask two brief questions to clarify two issues? What is poly-beta-hydroxybutyric acid, chemically speaking? In addition, I always see figures for protein which are just 6.25 times nitrogen. How much of that "protein" is actually protein? The most important question would be: How much of the nitrogen is nucleic acid?

CALLOWAY: That is a question I would also like to have the answer to. There have been some DNA determinations on the organism, but not any RNA analyses.*

The reason for our concern is uric acid formation. If the organism is anything like *E. coli* in its concentration of nucleic acid—13 percent of the dry solids—the kidney may be unable to clear the uric acid that would be an end product of a diet based largely on the high-protein bacterium.

Our analyses indicate that organisms grown in adequate media contain 12 to 14 percent of nitrogen and about 9 percent lipid. Digitonide-precipitable sterol is fairly low; vitamin A is nil; and alpha-tocopherol is reasonably high for a product of this kind—5.76 mg. per 100 g. of dry bacteria.

The only biological work we have done concerned protein quality. We found the nitrogen of boiled organisms to be 93 percent digestible. Biological value was 77 in an experiment in which casein also had a biological value of 77. Values were the same for organisms ruptured by high-frequency sound.

We have high hopes of feeding *Hydrogenomonas* for a few days to mice as their sole source of food, in order to do total carbon-nitrogen balances, but we have only a few grams of cells left. We have not yet had any high-lipid organisms to study, and we would very much like to, because we do not know whether the unusual lipid will be absorbable.†

K. SCHWARZ: What do you call poly-beta-hydroxybutyric acid? Is that a polyester, with ester linkage between the hydroxyl on one end and the carboxyl group on the next? This is the only way I could imagine it, but I do not think the name is a very good one, because it is not an acid any more.

BARNES: It is a polymer.

POLLARD: Is there another problem involved here also, in that in the usual diet of man you have such a heterogeneous source from which you

* Subsequent analysis by Mr. David Schwarz revealed 7.8 g. of nucleic acid per 100 g. bacterial dry solids, including 0.3 g. of DNA. Ed.

† We have since fed lipid-rich organisms to mice and found the lipid to be very poorly digested. Only about 15 percent was absorbed, but protein digestibility was the same as that of the protein-rich variety.

draw all your food, whereas here you are drawing your food from one source?

Is this going to induce a change in the bacterial flora of the host or interfere with some essential biochemical process in the host which you cannot readily detect? I wonder if a germfree animal might be useful for such studies. Minor differences might be magnified in a germfree animal which would be hidden in an animal supplied with microbial flora, which might supply that part which is missing.

JENKINS: As I mentioned earlier, I do not think that either these algal or bacterial systems will ever supply the major quantity of food for man, and it might be a relatively small part, and it might be important only for supplying the calories or specific components taken from them. So I do not know how important it is to study the details of whole cells fed 100 percent, and all that sort of thing.

BROBECK: I would like to suggest that one probably is going to have to do for these cultures what the dairy industry does for the fat in milk. The protein probably is going to have to be taken out and then added to the diet in whatever concentration you desire, rather than simply to plan to eat the unseparated organism the way it comes out of the culture.

D. SCHWARZ: This seems to me the preferred approach. Protein intake should be somewhere around 10 percent of diet dry solids in a formula diet. Here, you are dealing with organisms that may contain 70 percent protein. Some kind of balancing is obviously necessary.

In any case, if you want to make these biomasses more palatable, it is certainly feasible to fractionate them. Then you could achieve much more flexibility in your flavor mixes, and so forth.

We are doing this routinely in recovering biosynthesized radiochemicals by recovering from cells perhaps forty different components. Such components could be in balanced proportions.

KRAUSS: I suspect that if you can do this for *Hydrogenomonas*, you can certainly do it for *Chlorella*. It's no trick at all to shift the algae from 70 percent protein to 85 percent fat.

D. SCHWARZ: Well, I think to manipulate fat is less appealing from a technological standpoint than manipulating a carbohydrate of some kind and the protein. The fats are likely to give the most trouble. Can you increase the carbohydrate content? That's the question.

KRAUSS: Yes, you can. It is not as easy as increasing the fat.

K. SCHWARZ: You could make mutations and take strains which would probably produce much more carbohydrate.

BROBECK: It might turn out that instead of forcing the organism to produce a balanced diet, the easiest way to do this is to let the organism do what it can do easily, and separate the components and add the small amounts of the things you need to make it balance.

Acceptability of Biomasses as Food

BROWN: The question of acceptability has to be considered, and it may turn out that just for reasons of consumer acceptability one will find it is quite essential to process the raw algae or the raw bacteria by some other organism. It may turn out that this cannot be processed easily by nonbiological methods. I personally think this is wrong. I am very confident—and I am willing to bet at very large odds—that this is wrong; but I do not know for sure. It is a statement of faith.

I think that the matter is really important for a nonscientific reason. NASA is not going to fund bioregenerative systems adequately, I think, to get the hardware produced in time unless it is really convinced that this is the way to go. There is a fairly strong sentiment in many quarters to the effect that this is not the way to go, and it is based very largely on this intuitive feeling of the acceptability of these exotic foods.

The statement has been made that if it is feasible to feed the man what he is used to eating, we should not change it. If you examine this, it sounds very sensible, except that you know that there is a tremendous variation in what is acceptable. A great part of the population of the world lives on food that I myself would find rather unacceptable, if I had any choice, and at different stages in the development of the organism it goes through fads which to the adult seem unacceptable. (I remember for a very long time my son would eat anything, as long as it was spaghetti.)

We know that formula diets are adequate, or can be made adequate nutritionally for very long periods. It was pointed out that we all start life on a formula diet. Many experimental animals have been kept on formula diets as a routine—and this includes man.

I think the question of acceptability has been tremendously overrated. If I have a choice and if I can afford it, I am going to eat the kind of food I like, and if I do not have the choice, I will eat what is there, but I am surely going to eat if I can possibly stomach it. I know I need it. I am not particularly concerned about the taste, if I am desperate. If I am not desperate, I am very much concerned about the taste and about my particular mood, and I believe the astronauts are going to respond in much the same way.

Motivation, therefore, is clearly an important factor in what you call "acceptable." Also, the monotony of your experience is a factor. If you have nothing else to do except complain about the food or wish it were better, you are going to pay much more attention to it than if you are a busy man; and of course the duration of the experience is important.

If you have a reason, you can eat almost anything that provides the nutrition required. People have resorted to eating rats, which is generally considered unacceptable. They have also resorted to cannibalism, and other—shall we call them "exotic" foods?

Why do we then refuse to consider the possibility that the astronauts themselves could recognize that it was to their advantage to use food which was certainly not objectionable, but simply monotonous? But as long as you think you can have better food than that, you are going to insist on it.

I think in discussing the relative merits of these systems from the nutritional standpoint, all that we can really accomplish here is to identify for ourselves and perhaps for the record the salient problems—and it is clear that we are not going to get the answers. We do not have the backlog of experience on experimental animals or man fed bacteria or fed algae. What we do have is a clear demonstration of the engineering feasibility of producing foods of this sort.

However, let me emphasize again that the food is a minor part of the total engineering job, and it may well be that the decision of how to go will be made not on the food basis at all, but just on the gas management basis. End of speech.

BROBECK: Can I have time for rebuttal?

Yesterday, I said that I felt I was sitting through this movie a second time. I have heard this speech, practically word for word, on any number of occasions in connection with the World War II rations, including the episodic evidence about what people will eat under various conditions.

But I think the evidence is against the conclusion. Actually, it is impossible to overemphasize acceptability. The place where Allan and I agree is that formula diets are not unacceptable, and this is why this is one of the bright hopes of the future. It is not that they are unacceptable and adequate, but that they can be made acceptable and adequate. In the little paper I wrote on this I recommended very strongly that formula diets be used, not because they are unacceptable, but because they are acceptable.

I think it is a mistake to say that it is a question of acceptability versus adequacy. It is a question of both. The things have got to be adequate, but the men are not going to take them unless they are acceptable.

It seems to me the best illustration of this is what happened to margarine. You could ask the question: How cheaply do you have to sell margarine in order to compete with butter, if it is like the margarine on the market in 1935? The answer is: You cannot sell it cheap enough to make it compete. But when the margarine is altered so that it is practically indistinguishable from butter, then it has a great market.

I think the same principle applies to the use of these formula diets.

If it is a formula that tastes like algae, I am sure it will be unacceptable, but if it is a formula that tastes like a milkshake, then it may turn out to be a preferred food.

MAYER: I think one of the myths, of course, of nutrition is that food habits are fixed. Actually, even though the names of the foods have remained the same, a large proportion of the foods that are consumed by the American people are now different from the foods that were eaten a generation ago, and they keep on changing.

So I am not particularly concerned with whether the food is a usual food or not. I think that with highly motivated and selected and intelligent people this is a relatively easy problem, and I have great faith in what we can do now in terms of food technology, fragrance, and so on, so that it really is no great trick to make a diet moderately palatable, and particularly if it is going to be a fairly monotonous diet, it is not difficult to produce a small variety of flavors which can be mixed with the same base. I do not think this is the basic problem.

My feeling is that we know enough; and with due respect to Dr. Schwarz, I agree that there are probably factors that we do not know in human nutrition, or in mammalian nutrition at present, but I think that provided we take some insurance by not trying to do too pure a diet, we are unlikely to run into deficiencies in adults, as long as we are dealing with finite periods of one year, two years, and so on.

So it seems to me that the basic problems are not necessarily nutritional problems. The problems are problems of food processing and food technology, and I do not have the feeling at present that there is the effort in that area that is needed to explore the nutritional aspects of the various alternatives that Dr. Brown so ably mentioned.

BROWN: Would it be fair to say that if we consider the nutritional problems and the associated problems, that we have about the same amount of work to do if we decide to use conventional foods or formula diets?

TAPPEL: May I respond to that question of the food processing? It is often blocked out as "food processing" between the production of the bacteria and the feeding of the crew, as if this were a simple thing to do.

I think from the historical perspective of how this has taken place in the past we can gain a very valuable lesson. For example, let us just take the dehydrated food that is now being used in space missions and was produced as a military ration.

Its history dates back to World War I, and it was developed to a reasonable extent in World War II as a dehydrated food ration, and there were some hundred tons or so produced. It has come into production now as a freeze-dried component, but this has taken 15 years of research and development, and this is a very simple thing. Practically nothing was done to the starting material—conventional food—to get it up to this state of the art.

Let us take another simple one—or seemingly simple—that of radiation preservation, which was again aimed at a military ration, a ration for a selected group. Again the basic idea was just to kill the bacteria in the food to preserve the food—so it is very simple, really, and it involves only conventional foods, so there are no great innovations. This has progressed for 10 years, consumed many millions of research dollars, at one time had a hundred research groups operating on it, and still we do not have any of these developed to the practical state of use.

MAYER: What you are saying is that it is not the nutrition of man in space that we should be worrying about, but that it is the food technology of man in space, which is an entirely different thing.

TAPPEL: I am saying that we have the most unquantitative assessment of this.

MAYER: It may turn out in the long run, whether you are making food by this or that process, that the basic production of the food is of relatively little importance, at least for intermediary missions—six months to a year. Obviously, the longer you go, the greater your saving by adding a biological method, but nobody at present has any estimate of that missing component, which is the food processing factory between the algae or the bacteria and the astronaut.

JENKINS: This could be a very significant weight. The figures usually quoted I might add, are just the requirements for growing the organisms, and do not include the ancillary equipment of food processing and a number of other things—the CO_2 scrubbing, and all that sort of thing.

D. SCHWARZ: I think we are in a position to do a little thinking on that, because, in effect, we are getting components out of cells every day at about the scale that is required for maintaining a six- to ten-man daily mission. What is it? It is half a kilogram per man of solid food, or something like that; ten men—that is 5 kilograms a day.

This is not a huge factory. In fact, it does not have too much relation to mass production food technology. It has a lot more relationship to making fine chemicals.

MOSSEL: But you need solvents, and all that.

D. SCHWARZ: Sure! Nevertheless, you can reduce these to not too large units which are fairly easy to manage, and from our experience we would not predict that there would be a huge weight penalty.

HEGGENESS: Could you give some estimates, of the weight cost for the power as well as the factory?

D. SCHWARZ: We have not really attempted to do this. It might be useful to consider the composition and properties of some of these harvested cells (algae or *Hydrogenomonas*) in the light of our experience with certain other cells. Then, matching this against a model formula diet some picture of the equipment might emerge from which some initial estimates could be derived.

JENKINS: To terminate the discussion of the bioregenerative systems, I would like to read the statement by Dr. Bongers and Dr. Kok, relative to all of the bioregenerative systems, and particularly the *Hydrogenomonas*.

> "The bioregenerative systems are more or less in a transitory phase between research and development. The power data can be considered fairly accurate—at least within plus or minus 20 percent. The postulated weight data, however, represent approximations, particularly with respect to auxiliary equipment and construction materials. Also omitted are the weight penalties most probably involved in the processing of the solid output of the exchanges, elegantly defined as potential food. Further research is required in this area to evaluate the regenerative systems, especially the bacteria, with respect to this potential. Furthermore, as yet there is no experimental proof that the growth rates of the heavy bacteria suspensions can be realized in a large design to determine our relatively small scale with fairly precise control of physiological conditions and gas exchange. This aspect may affect considerably the weight involved in a chemosynthetic balanced system. Nevertheless, at present this approach still seems most promising."

I think that puts it in its proper context, that there is an awful lot yet to be done.

MAYER: What is too bad is that if we go to a wider human context than space, it may well be that unless we are more successful than we have been at managing the population of the earth, this is the one solid hope to avoid mass starvation, and therefore it is well worth putting a lot of resources into the food technology of algae and the food technology of microorganisms, and well worth a very major effort.

And yet this is, it seems to me, all the time the weakest component of any of our thinking on this.

VII. LAST WORDS

Discussion Leaders:

WALLACE O. FENN
Department of Physiology
University of Rochester
School of Medicine and Dentistry
Rochester, New York
and
H. N. MUNRO
Department of Biochemistry
University of Glasgow
Glasgow, Scotland

FENN: My notion about the program for this afternoon was to make it an opportunity for everybody or anybody, in addition to Dr. Munro, to have his last words, summarizing his own view on the subject; there may not be time enough for me to call on everybody. This session is not devoted to any one of the specific subjects which we have dealt with —it will be a general discussion of the whole substance of the Conference.

So without more ado I am going to ask Dr. Munro if he will give us his summation or his last words on this Conference.

MUNRO: Well, I hope they will not be my last words! To ask someone to summarize a conference—it just is not fair, you know.

Weight Penalties

The first question is: What about perspective? The thing I think we have to get quite clear is: What are the actual comparative relationships between the weights of materials to be flown into space and the various regenerative systems? Would regeneration become really important on the longer and more extensive missions? Would the present possibilities of power become quite critical at longer time intervals?

In other words, is power likely to develop more quickly than the speed of improvement in the yield of bioregeneration?

MAYER: It is perhaps the case that we have been too obsessed with problems of weight, and that the main use of bioregenerative systems in the long run may very well be in terms of Mars or moon colonies, much more than in problems of going there or coming back.

WARD: I agree fully, and I have almost limited my thinking to permanent planetary bases.

REYNOLDS: I wonder if the weight figures usually quoted are really comparable, since in the case of the dried food, one need not talk about a processing facility which must be included in the other systems.

JENKINS: The weight of the power unit required is not usually included either. Those figures are merely for producing the algae or the bacteria, so they are not comparable.

D. SCHWARZ: Somebody asked me to make a horseback figure to cover the food processing. If you want to put a weight per man in there, I would suggest you put 100 to 300 in as a starter.

JENKINS: To do what?

D. SCHWARZ: To convert the biomass to more usable food.

MUNRO: Two hundred kilograms per man?

D. SCHWARZ: Yes. But the weight per man will not be constant for any crew size because the basic process units for production for only one man would naturally be proportionately much higher. For this horseback number, I have assumed a ten-man crew, as suggested this morning. This must be taken as a very preliminary guess, but I think it bears some relation to reality.

MUNRO: I would suggest at this point that all we can do is to point to the dilemmas which will have to be resolved in the light of (a) improvement in thrust and (b) an estimate of the real cost of producing edible products from these bioregenerative systems.

REYNOLDS: I think you can always count on the fact that as long as it costs as much as it does to lift pounds away from the surface of the earth, pounds are going to be important. Just because you have a higher capability does not mean that you are ever going to want to use it less efficiently than you can.

ARNOLDI: May I supplement that remark by pointing out that even though a small percentage difference might not seem very significant, and it would always seem possible to design a booster which was 2 percent larger, the fact is that when you plan a specific mission you are confronted with a situation where a certain booster is available, and will be available on a certain schedule, and its capacity is fixed. Between the time that you decide upon the mission and try to select equipment for it there will be many second thoughts about what other devices or experiments you could take along, and at that point you begin to sort out the apples from the peaches and decide that you cannot afford the luxury of a one percent overweight life support system.

That is the point where weight becomes all-important, even down to the last ounce.

Nutrient Requirements

MUNRO: Well, that's the first dilemma, I think, the question of what system weights are in fact realistic.

The second question that struck me was our problem of nutrient requirements. Now, here there are, from the space point of view, two lots of nutrients. The nutrients are either macronutrients, in which case they weigh an appreciable amount, or they are micronutrients, where weight is not going to be a problem; but other factors enter in.

The questions are: What are the essential nutrients and how much? It is quite apparent that our knowledge of nutrient requirements at the minimum is still rather tenuous. However, the amount of knowledge varies with the different nutrients.

To begin with, with water and with calories—with energy—we can claim a fair degree of precision, and we can calculate the requirements for various tasks. In the case of these two nutrients, a reasonable estimate can be obtained.

In the case of protein we can obtain a reasonable order of magnitude. There are, as I have tried to indicate previously, various defects in our knowledge of protein requirements, but nevertheless the order of magnitude is probably 1 g./kg.

When we come down to the vitamins and the minerals, which will not appreciably contribute to the bulk, here we have factors and requirements which could be quite wildly out. We do not know precisely the amounts of some of the mineral and vitamin requirements, and we certainly have problems in knowing what factors may affect them. So you may say that it is adequate to give an excess.

Now, in the case of the vitamins, if you are dealing with the fat-soluble products, you will get toxicities; and in the case of the minerals, if you are loading up on these, you may have difficulties of interactions whereby, as we heard earlier, copper and zinc, for example, can give you an interaction whereby excess of one threatens the intake of the other.

So the net result is that precise and correct information must be provided on this topic.

Now, this is not merely important because of theoretical background. It is important because, if you are regenerating—recycling your water through ion exchange resins; if you are regenerating your food supply through a bioregenerative system, you may accidentally take out of your system minor components—particularly minerals—which will eventually over a long time interval show up as a deficiency. Therefore, the requirements here become potential hazards to long-term survival of man out in space.

The contingency requirements for space travel, of course, are unpredictable; that is, over and above the ones which are recognized from ordinary studies made on ordinary populations. Some of those which have come up are, first of all, calcium, and we really did not decide how to deal with this problem. Will fluoride of the order of 50 mg./day give you protection against loss from bed rest?

I mentioned a thought which is, perhaps, no more than a thought, that perhaps the effects on red cell production of protein level might be upset by space travel because of the effect of protein level on the hormone erythropoietin. This is merely a prediction of something to keep an eye on.

Thirdly, the emergence of new trace mineral deficiencies was suggested earlier, and this, of course, would crop up if the methods for purifying water or for bioregeneration resulted in the removal of substances the importance of which we do not yet know, and therefore one should be alive to this possible cause of trouble. All these points, and, I am sure, many others, demand continuous monitoring of any closed system which is devised.

Finally, we brought up the question of individual variation in requirements, and this might well be quite important. It is recognized not merely in the case of protein, which is where we discussed it, but also in the case of vitamin requirements. There are published data [106] showing the widespread needs by certain groups in the normal population, and it would certainly be unfortunate to include individuals with a higher requirement of any particular nutrient in a crew who were subsequently put into orbit.

These, then, are the points which I picked out in the question of supply of nutrients. I am not dealing now with problems of diet, which are really a separate question of how nutrients should be supplied. I wonder if there were some comments on this particular aspect which you would like to amplify.

Caloric Intake and Expenditure

BARNES: One of the things that was discussed was that we know very little about the influence of what might be considered suboptimal quantities of calories and perhaps other nutrients, including macronutrients—such as protein—on performance over long periods of time.

You have said that we can define the water and calorie requirements with precision. We can define requirements in terms of our normal living conditions under which we exist now, but perhaps we do not know the minimum under unusual conditions such as space travel.

MUNRO: You mean, in terms of survival? What can we tolerate?

BARNES: Well, stress and long-term performance. It has been pointed out that animals as well as humans may perform in certain respects better under conditions of what we would consider as slight deprivation in terms of common standards.

MAYER: It seems to me everybody has been very concerned with the possibility that people might not eat enough on the trip. I am a bit concerned, actually, with the opposite. Everything we know about the mechanism of regulation of food intake shows that, while by and large for normal animals and men it functions reasonably well in terms of adjusting intake to output, this is not the case when you go to either extreme; that is, either overexertion or underexertion.

We exercised rats on a treadmill for 20 minutes, 40 minutes, an hour, and so on, all the way up to eight hours. When we exercised the animals from one to six hours, their food intake did follow suit very well, and the animals' weight stayed constant. When you exercise them more, they eat more.

When you reach the level of exhaustion, of course, the food intake drops, and so does the body weight. We mentioned that earlier. This is what is observed in infantry on forced marches and situations of that sort.

The point that is of more concern with regard to the astronauts is that when you go below a certain level of energy expenditure, the voluntary food intake does not go down. In fact, it goes up, and it goes up in every species in which it has been tried; this is a phenomenon which farmers have known for centuries, which is why they coop up or pen up animals which they want to fatten, because the animals will eat as much —in fact, will eat somewhat more—than if they were going around on the range and as a result their weight will go up quite a bit.

A study I did in India showed very much the same phenomenon in an industrial population. If you have people who are reasonably active, they will exercise more, they will eat more, and their weight stays constant; but when you go into the inactive range, the food intake not only does not go down—it goes up, and the individuals become actually quite fat.

Now, it seems to me that among the things we should not forget are the normal risks to the human population. I know that there has been a tendency for medicine over the years to think in terms of: There are so many diseases, and once we have cured them there will be no more diseases. Actually, every time you change your environment, you change the nature of your diseases; and space, of course, creates all sorts of new problems in terms of radiation, problems of bacteriology, and so on and so forth.

We are dealing with a group of men, when we think of astronauts, for whom at present the first cause of death is coronary catastrophe. The second one is accident. It may very well be that in space we have different orders of priority; that accident is first, or, conceivably, that bacteriology comes back into its own. However, it seems to me that it would be imprudent to think in terms of trips of two or three years' duration, and neglect to think of what we can do in terms of nutritional prevention of the most prevalent cause of death for people at that age group.

Here we have a group of men who are at least at various times under stress, who are very inactive, and therefore likely to become obese, particularly if they have the wrong type of genetic constitution. I think that some attention ought to be paid to whatever we know in terms of nutritional prevention of coronary catastrophe, not only during the trip, but a long time before the trip.

It would be obviously a considerable problem to have somebody get a coronary on the way up or down, and anything that can be done to prevent it is important, and the problem of calories is closely related to it. I do not think that we can blindly assume that the caloric adjustment will be automatic, and that if people are presented the food, they not only will eat enough of it, but that they will eat too much of it.

MUNRO: You can, of course, control this better in a population in space than you can ever hope to do in the general population.

POLLARD: If you have a bioregenerative system, you could attune that to consumption.

MAYER: Yes. I think we also have to be prepared, though, for the fact that the astronauts may be constantly hungry. You see, when you get below that level of energy expenditure, you have people who may be constantly slightly hungry, and this is something that ought to be taken into consideration.

FENN: I think it might be important to know how far you can stretch a limited food supply. I wondered what the curve would be if you tried to plot survival time against calorie intake. I mean, 100 calories a day—how much would that prolong your life if you had to get home and you were running out of food? How much would 100 calories a day prolong your life? How much would 200 do, or 500, and so on?

I do not know that there are any data on this.

MUNRO: I think the survival rations have been studied by Johnson,[107] particularly.

CALLOWAY: Not in terms of survival, though, Dr. Munro.

MUNRO: In terms of effects on the individuals; not in terms of human survival.

FREMONT-SMITH: There would need to be survival with some degree of effectiveness—being able to function at least on a minimal level.

FENN: You would have to be able to lie down when you decelerated, and some manipulation of the apparatus would probably be essential.

Food Forms

MUNRO: This certainly is a point; namely, that what is survival on earth may not be compatible with operating instrumentation under space travel. In other words, the psychological effects may be unfavorable, sufficiently so to be serious. This we do not know.

Now, the third point which emerged was the diversity of food supply. There are some general points which occurred to me.

First of all, we have the possibility of using natural foods, and here it seems mandatory to have them dehydrated, purely from a point of view of weight. However, here the questions are ones of food technology, and it was emphasized that storage problems and antioxidant additions were important in obtaining a product which would also keep.

The second alternative is the formula diet, and this, we saw, is quite a problem to manipulate. First of all, the data which were presented by Mr. David Schwarz demonstrated that people can in fact live on chemically defined formula diets, and this, I think, is a very important positive gain. An experiment can be done with a formula diet over a long period.

The advantages which came out were, first of all, a low residue—low fecal output—which would be desirable; secondly, the blood cholesterol level was reduced, and this might be relevant to the question of long-term survival in the face of potential coronary disease.

There are some points which were not discussed which might be serious. The free amino acids may give rise to an intestinal upset. They may affect your bacterial population in the gut, and I do not remember whether anybody mentioned this possibility, but perhaps you would like to make a comment on this at this stage.

Have you any predictions to make from this type of formula diet? Will it alter the flora?

GUSTAFSSON: It will alter the flora to begin with, but if you continue on these formula diets, whether they are these very sophisticated ones that you are employing or the semisynthetic diets we are using in animal experiments, you get a situation of steady state, where you can control the whole thing. You know what you have, and you know pretty well that if you do not change anything the flora will keep fairly constant. I think you should not forget to include among these formula diets also the less expensive diets—what I call semisynthetic diets—which we have been using for many years in animal experiments. They are very easy to make. We know very much about them in all kinds of animal experiments, and they could be brought down to the same bulk as the synthetic ones. And they keep in a dry state as well as the others.

K. SCHWARZ: I would like to mention one other advantage of a formula diet which is very considerable, and that is, as soon as you recognize a special need for additional amino acids or one specific amino acid, for a trace element or for a vitamin, the lacking substance can easily be added. This may be much more difficult if you have natural foods.

MUNRO: But you hope not to recognize that during the space mission?

K. SCHWARZ: No, but since the space mission will probably lead to unanticipated stress situations and requirements which we cannot really foresee, this potential should not be neglected.

MUNRO: It can be considered the other way round; namely, that the natural food has a better chance of containing the materials to meet this special, previously unrecognized hazard.

K. SCHWARZ: Not necessarily. Foods as we get them today—and as they may be in these dehydrated sandwiches that are suggested for space travel—may be limited in a number of things. Marginal deficiencies may come up.

MUNRO: Would this not be covered by supplementation of the natural diet, if you added supplementary sources?

K. SCHWARZ: Well, then you are in a formulation.

POLLARD: Dr. Munro, I would like to ask if anyone has studied the variability of man's requirements in relation to his intestinal flora. We know that there are some organisms that contribute to the diet, and there are some that delete from the diet. Would it be worthwhile to standardize the intestinal flora of the individuals who are going to be involved in such a flight, so that you could at least get a baseline which would have some relevance to the problem of dietary sufficiency?

MUNRO: This is true of the B complex of vitamins, where a considerable part of the complex is provided from intestinal sources, but it can also, equally, be supplied from the exterior.

MAYER: One advantage of the formula diet, outside of the fact that one could stabilize people on it, probably, more easily, is that it would allow for a more precise definition or prescription of how many calories somebody ought to have.

Now, perhaps I am obsessed by this, and perhaps it seems unrealistic, but I would simply like to point out that a pound of fat—an extra pound of body fat—is roughly the equivalent of 3500 calories. That means that if an individual is systematically eating 100 calories more a day than he is expending, which is perhaps only 3 or 4 percent, or 2 percent, of his requirements, in one month this is a pound of fat; in a year this is 12 pounds of fat.

How is he going to know that he is gaining quite a bit of fat? He cannot weigh himself in the capsule, and he is an active man gaining weight fairly rapidly without too many ways of knowing it.

There are some advantages, if we want him still to be able to get into his tight-fitting space suit, to really know fairly adequately what the caloric requirements of this particular astronaut are when he is essentially inactive in a capsule, and it is very much easier to tell him to eat that much and no more if you are feeding him a formula diet, than if he is juggling with dehydrated apricots, or all sorts of other more succulent foods that are prepared for him by the Quartermaster Corps.

FENN: What difference does it make if he stored it as fat or stored it in the cupboard? It is about the same weight either way, and he can still use it.

ARNOLDI: From an engineering point of view, a space suit is a carefully tailored device, and if you change your actual physical volume, or the proportions of your body, it undermines the usefulness of the space suit in an emergency.

I am not talking about growing so fat that you cannot put it on any more, but simply changing your proportions relative to the carefully tailored proportions of the suit.

MAYER: I think it is very easy for a good, mesomorphic, previously active individual in a small space to put on 20 pounds in a year.

MUNRO: This merely emphasizes that body weight has to be controlled. It has to be controlled, presumably, on the basis of the caloric intake.

RAHN: It might be possible to weigh the man in space. I think on prolonged missions we may have to do that by producing small accelerations and measuring these known impacts, which allows us to calculate the mass.

REYNOLDS: What he may have to do is put on enough fat to make up for the loss in muscle mass.

MUNRO: Even Shakespeare had this problem, you remember, where in *Midsummer Night's Dream* he talks about Puck, who says, "I'll throw a girdle round the earth"—which is more or less a space-containment problem.

CALLOWAY: People will adapt to a surprisingly wide range of caloric intakes. We have tried manipulating body weight of experimental subjects by changes in caloric intake and by changes in physical work, within a fairly narrow range. Subjects will maintain constant body weights regardless of whether you make them do an hour's more work on a treadmill a day, or whether you take away 200 calories from the diet.

Our subjects have rarely maintained absolute body composition, in spite of the fact that for 90 days body weight was nearly constant. I would question Dr. Munro's statement that we can specify caloric needs.

K. SCHWARZ: I would like to point out and emphasize that gravity may have a lot to do with the regulation of bone growth and of calcium and phosphorus metabolism. Very interesting work by Becker and others recently has proven that gravity or other stress is effective in micro-systems, by way of semiconductor effects, in regulating bone growth and removal of bone tissue. Becker[108] has found that one can treat these microscopic elements of bone as semiconducting feedback mechanisms which control bone structure. Gravity exerts mechanical stress like any other pull or pressure. Through a biological transducer (apatite-collagen positive-negative junction) this stress is converted into a significant biological signal which in turn, through a second biological transducer (orientation and alignment of collagen fibers), leads to oriented bone growth. It is quite possible that similar systems also enter into the regulation of growth of muscle, elastic tissue, the cardiovascular system, or even the kidney or the brain.*

RAHN: Do you think it might have an effect upon the redistribution of fat in the body?

K. SCHWARZ: Yes, and upon just how much fat there is. We have heard about the redistribution of calcium. Why not also fat?

REYNOLDS: I was thinking of all these people with fat shoulders.

CALLOWAY: I never knew it was gravity that caused the observable change from sitting in a chair.

K. SCHWARZ: There may be another minor factor about the formula diet. If you are going to buy a regenerator, then you eliminate all the problems of storage and stability.

Secondly, if you separate the ingredients, you also simplify greatly the storage stability, because you don't have interactions.

Bioregenerative System Stability

MUNRO: The other systems are bioregeneration and the possibility of chemical synthesis. I wonder, in the case of bioregeneration, whether there is any evidence of genetic change in your organism. Is there a possibility that any of the systems so far suggested may in fact alter genetically during the course of prolonged regeneration and develop different properties?

KRAUSS: I would comment very briefly on that. We have observed in the long-term cultures that there are readjustments in the metabolism of the organism—some readjustments in growth rate, some adjustments in analytical levels—but I should say, in general, that whatever genetic drift there is develops in favor of increased production. Those mutants which cannot keep up with the so-called wild type, the original type, do

* Extensive discussion of this topic will be found in Volume II of this series. Ed.

tend to fall out. I would be very much surprised to see a genetic drift which reduced production.

However, a genetic drift which might bring about a change in the analytical composition of the organism which was unexpectedly damaging but not inhibitory to growth as such is always possible. Experiments to try to verify this might well be performed.

MAYER: What about the drift that would create a new nutritional requirement for the organism, as has happened when you bombard neurospora and produce arginine-dependent neurospora, and so forth.

KRAUSS: Yes, but in a large culture with many millions of organisms, those tend to pass out of the system. They wash out, and those that are not so damaged survive.

RAHN: Dr. Krauss, I heard you use the phrase "wild type." Is this the way you regard genetically your culture? Is it a wild type?

KRAUSS: Let us say, original type. We have used many cultures, but most of those which we use are types which have been isolated from nature.

FREMONT-SMITH: Originally—at least at one point.

WARD: It should be pointed out, of course, that these are asexually reproducing organisms. If you go through a unialgal isolation and obtain a clone from a single cell, then theoretically you should have a genetically stable population. Of course, you could get minor genetic fluctuations due to spontaneous mutation.

RAHN: In other words, this is what we would be considering, and it would obviously be minor and of no concern.

POLLARD: Dr. Rahn, there was a reference to that this morning, that a system could be regenerated in hours.

WARD: Reseeded in hours, sure. As Dr. Brown, I think, pointed out, it is probably quicker to do that than to clean the equipment.

POLLARD: Can they be lyophilized to provide starter cultures?

WARD: Algae have been lyophilized. Not with a high degree of success, I do not believe, but they have been lyophilized.

BROWN: Some can.

KRAUSS: The blue-greens can.

REYNOLDS: What is the possibility of a culture becoming sick from some mechanical defect in the system and producing toxic products which are not recognized in time to keep from including them in your process?

FREMONT-SMITH: Or by virus infection and transduction, which is certainly not eliminated in any of our considerations here. We have not been able to deal with the viruses, and we know very well that a virus can cause a very definite mutation and an entirely different organism as to characteristics.

WARD: It is quite possible that algal cultures could become contaminated with toxic materials as a result of mechanical breakdown of accessory pieces of equipment such as fuel cells, light sources, etc. A wide variety of materials commonly used in space crafts are known to be toxic to algae.

A point of interest that I did not mention this morning is that algal cultures, like germfree animals, are either completely free of contaminants or are heavily contaminated. For example, if you start an algal mass culture using axenic algae, sterile inorganic medium, and sterile culture apparatus and do not protect completely from invasion of other micro-organisms, you will soon have a high contaminant population. Depending on the steady-state algal mass, bacterial populations can range from 10^4 to 10^7 viable cells/ml. of algal culture.

BROWN: Would you care to make a judgment or hazard a guess as to which would be the better way to go in algal cultures—keep them aseptic, or deliberately keep them contaminated? I know you cannot answer, but you can guess.

WARD: If I have to guess, I would say that contaminated cultures would be the most practical. I say this because axenic cultures are extremely difficult to maintain, at least on a large scale. Maintenance of contaminant-free algal mass cultures would require complete biological separation between man and his life support system as well as sterility of almost the entire spacecraft, including electronic components. Sooner or later I would expect crosstransfer or bacterial contamination of the algal culture. Bacterial contaminants survive and multiply very well on excretory products of algae. Unfortunately, in one of our recent studies we found that some enteric pathogens not only survive, but multiply in algal cultures. Most human pathogens would not survive due to their rather strict metabolic requirements.

KRAUSS: I think there is also another aspect to this problem. I am not sure I completely agree with Dr. Ward with regard to the advisability of trying to keep a culture sterile. It can be done. It takes some doing.

However, it may be in the long run that the choice of an organism will be dictated by its ability to survive well and produce well in the presence of contaminating organisms—a criterion which has scarcely been touched upon in the consideration of the various candidates for this kind of system.

POLLARD: As a bacteriologist I would be opposed to this. I shudder at the thought of mixed cultures under conditions that you cannot anticipate.

MOSSEL: And what happens if your system is not entirely protected against invasion from the outside, and if *Staphylococcus aureus* or a man's *Klebsiella aerogenes* would grow—

POLLARD: You could pollute the air.

MOSSEL: You would pollute the air; you would pollute the food; this might give rise to the formation of toxins—and this is really dangerous.

K. SCHWARZ: And molds also.

WARD: You have a point there. However, I should like to cite an observation that Dr. James E. Moyer and I made several years ago when we first started working on the contaminants of algal cultures. We collected samples of the same alga from mass cultures being grown in eight different laboratories scattered throughout the United States. With only minor modifications, the same bacterial contaminants were isolated from each of the cultures. Most cultures had significant populations of only five or six different bacteria, which means that the types of bacteria that can multiply in algal cultures are fairly limited.

FREMONT-SMITH: But you did not mention *Staphylococcus*.

WARD: That is true and it could get into an algal culture, but it probably would not survive. A contaminated steady-state algal culture is a fairly stable ecological system. Organisms with higher competitive advantage predominate, while others generally die out. We have found that most contaminant bacteria that can flourish in algal cultures without competition generally die out when in competition with other more competitive microorganisms. Hence, it might be better to deliberately contaminate with highly adapted harmless bacteria than to have the algal system subject to overrun by a pathogen that can only survive without competition.

MOSSEL: This may be enough of a safety valve under the conditions on earth, but I would shiver to be the microbiologist to give the advice: Go ahead with this mixed culture. And I think that all of us microbiologists would join with me in that.

POLLARD: Has the algal food been tested exhaustively as far as adequacy is concerned?

WARD: Not at all.

POLLARD: So you are not even sure that the food is sufficient qualitatively.

WARD: This is quite true, and I am sure from past studies that the bacteria present have influenced the quality and acceptability of the algal products used.

POLLARD: So, actually, at the present time you are on more secure ground with your formula diet, and yet the bioregenerative system has been going longer than the organized program for a formula diet?

WARD: Oh, no. I do not think this is true. The formula diets have been used for years.

BARNES: There is the matter of bioregeneration in order to take care of wastes and in order to provide oxygen. I do not think anyone here has talked about food from algae as being the sole source of food. They have only talked about it as being a minor component.

MOSSEL: Even a minor component of the diet may be quite dangerous when it becomes contaminated.

May I ask a question? With this *Hydrogenomonas* we bacteriologists have had very little experience, but we know that it is related to some nonpigmented *pseudomonas* species, which may be rather toxic. Unless you protect your culture here and make it free from any contaminants, I think you should not even consider it.

POLLARD: One of our major problems in our animal colonies when we are doing radiation work is *pseudomonas.* It can knock out experiments completely.

KRAUSS: I will not dispute the desirability or the possibility of an aseptic culture of these organisms. There is one thing, however, that is advantageous when dealing with algal cultures. These grow in inorganic media, you remember. They are not glucose media, or anything of the sort.

The microbial population that exists there is existing on whatever products are secreted by the organisms during normal culture, and this is at a reasonably low level. This does, of course, depend somewhat upon the strain and the conditions, but one does have something working for him with regard to keeping bacterial contamination down in cultures of this sort.

K. SCHWARZ: But it is not the amount, but the quality of the bacterial contamination which counts. If you have one pathogenic organism in there, and it starts multiplying just a little bit, you are through if you get that into the human.

MOSSEL: And also under terrestrial conditions this may be true, but what if for some reason the autolysis in this culture increases in your algae? You have organic material shed—voided—into the medium, and immediately any potential pathogen will use this opportunity—

KRAUSS: This is true of any perishable food source.

MOSSEL: I agree entirely.

MUNRO: To what extent would it be necessary in these bioregenerative systems to have to carry a trained member of the crew who knew how to manipulate them? Would you be adding to your passenger load?

BROWN: No, this is easy.

Could I also register an objection as to the basis of making a decision about sterile versus contaminated cultures? I do not know myself whether I agree that one should not think about contaminated cultures, but I think this is a debatable point and there are arguments on both sides.

The important factor is the stability of the culture. The possible sources of trouble can and should be examined. I do not think intuition is any criterion here.

FREMONT-SMITH: Should you not say, then, not a "contaminated" culture, but a specified mixed culture? Because a contaminated culture means just a bunch of unknowns, and then I think we are really in trouble.

BROWN: An unknown mixed culture which, at any time, you could analyze to determine what the constituents are, if you wanted to do the work—this is precisely what I mean. The composition may change with time, and I would expect it to change within certain ranges, but the mixture itself is likely to be reasonably stable, because the conditions, ecologically speaking, are pretty restricted.

However, I would be not at all hopeful that one could insert a series of organisms and say: This is what it is going to be. You would have to allow for the automatic self-regulating mechanisms.

The only thing you can be sure you have is a single organism, if you choose to go that route. Once you start forgetting about the precautions and allow some contamination to get in, then you no longer have control over that. I think it is a choice between a single organism or an unprotected system, or an inadequately protected system.

FREMONT-SMITH: You think the ecological constancy is more important than a single organism? I see the point.

GUSTAFSSON: May I add from years of experience—that it is as difficult to keep a normally germfree isolator unit as a noncontaminated, large-scale, pure culture for a long period of time. One has to have exactly the same technical outfit and standards in both instances.

However, I hope I do not misunderstand Dr. Brown. You are talking about an open culture, where you hope that your algae themselves produce conditions that keep out other microorganism?

BROWN: You cannot avoid having that situation. This is exactly what you will have, if you do not take precautions.

GUSTAFSSON: Yes, but I am not so sure that you will have that because even if the algae has the chair, so to say, all the other contaminants will be there to a certain extent and in varying amounts and of different types. In an open system, you will from time to time get in new contaminants, and it will take some time until they disappear again, and during that time they might cause endless disturbances in the product form.

BROWN: The point that I think we are overlooking is that when you have a large enough system, it has a kind of stability that a test-tube system does not have. It tends to resist a foreign contaminant coming in.

There is a range of fluctuation possible, of course, but I think the possible population compositions are much less than the mathematically possible ones.

GUSTAFSSON: Well, take a cow, for example, that has a continuous culture of 300 l. maximum to 100 l. minimum. That can change very easily, resulting in bloating and the death of the animal.

Man has about 2 kg. of culture all the time in his bowel, which is changing according to diet and other not too well known factors. It is not so bad for the man, however, because it is down in the bowel where you do not absorb too much except water. Your culture is to be used as food, however, and whatever you have accidentally got into your system will eventually be absorbed by the astronaut.

CALLOWAY: I would like to ask about urine as a growth medium. Suppose something happens and they all start pumping out unusual amounts of hormone, or something like that. What does that do to the organism that you are growing on a urine substrate?

REYNOLDS: There was one point made that I would like to respond to. Dr. Ward mentioned the electronic components not being sterilizable.

WARD: With difficulty.

REYNOLDS: Well, I think it is important to note, though, that for the sterilization requirement on planetary missions a large number of electronic components are now being selected or developed to have the required high reliability after undergoing sterilization cycles, and so I think that possibly with a few exceptions these things will be available off the shelf in a few years, and the few that would be a problem could be readily taken care of.

K. SCHWARZ: I would like to refer to Dr. Pollard's last comment. I do not think that it is the simple problem: Is the biomass per se a good food? I think the problem is: Is the biomass a good raw material to make a food or a portion of a food? That is the point, and that is a more complicated problem to study, but that is the way it ought to be studied, in my opinion.

BARNES: There is another question that has been on my mind relating to toxicity. The studies that have been done with the algae mass in feeding experiments, I gather, have been with algae that have been cultured under air—that is, 80 percent nitrogen. Is there any difference in the algae and their components when you culture under pure oxygen at one-third atmosphere? Has this ever been studied?

KRAUSS: Algae have been studied under quite a different number of atmospheres—argon-supplanting nitrogen; various levels of oxygen, etc.

One thing we can say is that elevated levels of oxygen do reduce photosynthesis and reduce algal growth—that is, oxygen levels above the normal 20 percent in air.

BROWN: Since oxygen is being produced photosynthetically, would you want to guess how much oxygen is elevated in the usual culture?

KRAUSS: This depends so much. We have just finished a whole series of studies on how fast you have to sweep the oxygen out to get over this. I do not have those data with me, but there is a marked increase.

BROWN: I would like a ballpark figure, because I am sure you are well over 21 percent in the average culture that has been studied.

KRAUSS: I do not disagree with the fact that it must be elevated to some degree, but I suspect it is not a great deal, because of the rate of sweep we normally employ in order to get the CO_2 in to maintain your steady state photosynthesis.

RAHN: The question is: What is your pO_2 in the algal culture?

KRAUSS: It depends upon the temperature of the algae culture.

RAHN: On a typical run?

WARD: In our machines it runs around 200 mm.

MUNRO: Has anyone tried growing algal cultures at 5 lb. to the square inch in pure oxygen?

WARD: We have grown a few cultures in flasks. We have varied the total pressure and partial pressures of carbon dioxide, oxygen, and nitrogen. Most of this work was done by Dr. S. S. Wilks at the USAF School of Aerospace Medicine at Brooks AFB. However, I do not believe the results are quantitative enough for publication yet. I do not have the gadgetry to run a steady-state algal culture under reduced pressure.

BROWN: Is short-term growth possible at these reduced pressures?

WARD: Oh, yes.

MAYER: I think Dr. Pollard's point needs to be amplified. I think that from everything we know there is no reason to think that any protoplasm, properly processed, could not be a source of food, particularly if it has enough carbohydrate.

On the other hand, it seems quite obvious from what we have said earlier that you are going to be left with quite a lot of material which you do not want. For instance, you will be left with a lot of chlorophyl, or maybe left with a lot of purines and pyrimidine and nucleic acid. So I think that one of the assumptions we should not make is that all of the food that we produce is going to go round and round in the man. We have spoken a great deal about the fact that the food may need to be supplemented, but we have not said anything about the fact that a great deal of the production might have to be rejected and either chewed up by a different type of bacteria or burned or otherwise put back into the cycle through a nonhuman intermediary.

WARD: There is always the possibility that rejected protoplasm, that not used, can be put through the waste disposal system and eventually recycled.

D. SCHWARZ: This raises the question of whether it is easier to handle waste disposal from a processing standpoint external to the man, or whether you want to deal with the man's waste.

If you feed him the whole cell, for example, then he digests it, and you have got his fecal output to deal with. If you feed him only selected portions of it, then you have the waste products of the food processing step, and that might be a little bit easier to control.

MAYER: If you were to feed him all of this, you might end up with a very gouty astronaut.

POLLARD: I am really concerned, though, about this open system that you are talking about. Let me give you an example of what I mean.

I worked in a laboratory in which *Brucella* vaccine was being produced. This is a human pathogen. Therefore, the organisms were kept under very stringent control. However, anyone who was infected with *Brucella,* or sensitized to *Brucella,* immediately had a headache as soon as he entered the building.

There were no viable *Brucella* floating around in that laboratory. If you intend to expose a man for 16 months to a *Chlorella* environment, is there any possibility that he might become so sensitive to *Chlorella* that it would be toxic to him?

K. SCHWARZ: That is another point, I think.

MOSSEL: And a very important one, I think.

KRAUSS: He becomes so sensitive to *Chlorella* that—what? That he might manifest some anaphylactic or sensitivity phenomena to it?

MUNRO: This all emphasizes the question of the unknown factors.

It seems to me that one of these is the question of how long it will take eventually to develop this bioregenerative system, assuming that no major snags occur in relation to the times required to mount the project which will require such a system.

Do the people working in this field think that most of these things can be cleared up in, let us say, five years?

MAYER: It seems to me every single one of those questions could be answered here on earth.

K. SCHWARZ: Or at least in an orbiting space laboratory.

MAYER: Oh, no. It could be answered here.

K. SCHWARZ: Not necessarily. We have to get away from gravity, I think.

KRAUSS: Well, one thing that I think is emerging from this discussion, is that this is indeed a difficult problem and a most enormously complex problem. The level of effort required to do a thing of this sort is very high regardless of which organism one is choosing.

MUNRO: Another question which we have not considered very much, really, but which is brought up by the fourth source of potential food supplies—chemical synthesis, from, say, methane to carbohydrate—is: What proportion of the total load will be provided by bioregeneration or chemical synthesis, or can we have a mixed system, or alternatively, will the system vary according to where the astronaut is, traveling or located in his final station?

What are the implications from the experts on bioregeneration about setting up algal cultures on other planets? Will this give you greater stability?

KRAUSS: Well, it could give greater stability, but whether you have greater stability in the system is always a question.

I think one of the problems that one faces in looking at a closed ecology is the fact that you sacrifice stability when you restrict the number of organisms. You have got theoretically one man and one microorganism of some sort. On this planet the balance is reasonably stable, because there is a very large and complex system supporting both segments of the economy. Now we are trying to engineer this down and compress it to a stable system with just two organisms—or perhaps two or three organisms. I think the problem of whether one can indeed efficiently engineer stability into the system or not is the basic problem, whether on another planet or in a space vehicle.

MUNRO: You might, of course, choose to have your space vehicle entirely supplied by dehydrated natural foods, and your planet supplied partially by bioregeneration. The choices may not be absolute ones.

FENN: Dr. Munro, how are you getting along with your summary? We have interrupted you so much, and you have asked to be interrupted so many times, that I am not sure whether you are just beginning or just ending.

MUNRO: I am merely regurgitating bits and pieces that were only partially digested during the course of the discussion.

I wish I were a ruminant.

The next question which we considered, since the Chairman has tactfully reminded me to continue with this, is the question of acceptability. The first point which was considered, I think, was whether the natural diet is the easiest one to accept. There seems to be a general feeling that people did not change very readily.

The second point was that if the formula diet is produced, then you have to do something to it to make it acceptable.

And the third point which I think we came to was that individual variation in tolerance to unusual foods is quite considerable, and that a selection based on this of suitable subjects might well be advantageous.

Are there any afterthoughts on this particular problem? Because, obviously, this is closely tied up with the question of algal cultures, with intermediates through which these products might be passed in order to produce a palatable food, whether it is worth even attempting to feed human subjects for part of the time directly on algal or bacterial materials.

TAPPEL: I think we want to take the long perspective relative to formula diets and algal diets, and so forth, and as has been brought out here now, when these are brought under intellectual discussion, Scientist A will bring up Objection A, and this has to be investigated in great detail. So once you go through Scientists A to Z and all of these questions—which are really valid questions—you have ahead of you a formidable amount of research; whereas with the present military rations now available, you not only know something about the acceptability, you not only have great variety, but you can also predict from the past experience of the people using them what they would like.

It seems to me that the choice is one of having a very vast scientific study of other choices, which I hope does develop, because this would be good for society—but you have to take a very long view of this, and we always have the present rations to fall back on, which I will predict we will be using 10, 15, 20 years from now.

MUNRO: The other aspect which was mentioned as well was, of course, the problem of rhythms and frequency of meals, the changes in the natural circadian rhythm, the changes in the number of meals offered to the subjects. These are probably relatively minor points, once the major one of acceptability is dealt with.

Germfree Astronauts

And then the final aspect which we dealt with—not the final in point of time, but the last one which I have summarized here—is the effect on the intestinal population. As you may remember, the object which we eventually came down to was to maintain normal flora, and this suggested that one might even carry a stock of normal flora to reinoculate the subject. I think that was suggested at one point.

POLLARD: What is a "normal flora"?

MUNRO: Perhaps Dr. Gustafsson would help out with that query.

GUSTAFSSON: I agree with Dr. Pollard. We discussed yesterday that we do not know what is a normal flora.

If a man is going on a long mission, and he is preconditioned and seems to be in good health and in good spirits, I would suggest that you take the bacterial flora that he has at that time and try to conserve that one way or another, to feed back to him, so to say, later on.

MAYER: Short-circuiting the recycling.

GUSTAFSSON: This is the only answer we can give today, until we know better what are the necessary constituents of a normal flora. Do you not agree with that, Dr. Pollard?

POLLARD: Well, here again you have such a big mixture. I would like to know exactly what organisms you feel are essential for man. There are some organisms which he can do without. So, therefore, I would be more selective and say that there are perhaps eight or nine organisms with which man should be seeded that are essential to his well-being.

We have established a defined flora in some of our germfree animals. We are studying the population dynamics within this enclosed environment to see what the fluctuations in microbial population would be in time, and what the fluctuations would be in relation to diet. These, I think would provide us with more precise information than to just take his flora—many of the organisms would not even survive—and feed them back to him.

In fact, I would be more inclined to give a defined flora, one which would be beneficial to the man.

GUSTAFSSON: I am sorry you were not here yesterday when I suggested that we should have a minimum flora, which is what you are talking about, and I said something to the effect that: If you are putting this all the way out to the last, final conclusion, it is easier to keep the man germfree, because the germfree state plus a well-defined diet is easier to maintain, maybe, than an animal or man with a flora.

POLLARD: We do not know. There may be some very labile food constituents derived from organisms which a defined diet, or a chemically defined diet, may not contain.

GUSTAFSSON: But I was using your finding in this conclusion, that you have been able to raise mice for three generations on a very well-defined formula diet.

POLLARD: However, they are stunted. They have trouble getting off the ground, and we have some distance to go yet before we feel that the diet is comparable to that in the conventional animal.

You know, you cannot extrapolate information from mice to man, and a diet that may be quite adequate in mice may not be very good for man. So while we may work out a wonderful chemically defined diet in mice and in rats, I do not know how we can do the same thing in man.

WARD: Well, I will tell you what: You sterilize the man and eliminate all the problems associated with his microflora, and we will take care of the algae and keep them free from microorganisms.

RAHN: I have a technical question. How do you reinoculate a man? Can you do it per os, or will they be destroyed?

GUSTAFSSON: No. You have the microorganisms in a capsule that is not digested in the stomach; it is digested further down.

BROWN: I understand that there are cases where it is very difficult to reestablish a flora, and I have no idea whether these are exceptions or whether this is what you might expect in many cases.

GUSTAFSSON: I think they have not given enough inoculation material to these patients. If you give a small amount of a bacterium or a mixed population of bacteria, it cannot establish itself due to the fact that other strains hold the ground and are producing antibiotic substances, and what-not.

K. SCHWARZ: Can you give us quantities? What do you call a rather large or small amount?

GUSTAFSSON: Five or 10 g. in man.

POLLARD: We just pour a culture of it on the food and the animals eat it.

GUSTAFSSON: How sure are you that it gets in?

POLLARD: They eat it.

MOSSEL: But how can you be sure that it gets where it should go, into the ileocecal region; that it is not partly killed off, by the gastric barrier and, hence, never gets a chance to influence the bacterial population of the ileocecal region.

POLLARD: Well, we have not had any trouble with it. We have six organisms—

MOSSEL: In man?

POLLARD: I am not talking about man. I do not know anything about man.

FENN: Dr. Mossel, do you have anything to add?

MOSSEL: The only thing is, that if we are considering giving lyophilized bacterial cultures, as a drug or as a corrective measure on these space flights, we should in all detail study what numbers of organisms we begin with and what numbers of organisms we find at a given moment. In other words, we shall have to know what the stability of the organisms in those capsules is. In the little bit of work that we have done in "implantation therapy," as it is called in Great Britain, we have found that you may very well start out with gelatin capsules containing ten to the twelfth per gram of substance of *L. acidophilus* or *B. bifidus* or *Ristella,* or whatever you want to apply; but that, just by storage at room temperature, or even under refrigeration, you lose your organisms at a high rate, and this is for known organisms.

So I would like to underline that if it is decided by the top brass to use this method, some research is highly needed so as not to have the happy illusion that we are administering bacteria, when in fact we are giving almost nothing else than a neutral filler.

Well, I think with that the subject has been well covered.

LIVINGSTON: Mr. Chairman, I learned for the first time at this meeting that it might be practicable to get a germfree man. If this is feasible, why not have the whole capsule germfree, except for whatever plants you might want to have for bioregenerative systems? Then you do not have to worry about your food being sterilized; you do not have to worry about food spoilage, and you do not have to worry about contaminating bioregenerative cultures. The astronaut can presumably do anything he wants in the system and not upset it.

BROWN: How are you going to get him back?

LIVINGSTON: Oh, you would have to debrief him, including a bacteriological reintroduction, but if he is going to be gone for three years, after all, I should think that might be feasible to think about.

Authorities have spoken with concern about contaminating the planets; this would provide a way to insure that contamination could not occur.

I had always assumed that you could not arrange for a germfree man; but Professor Gustafsson has suggested you can. It seems to me that maybe a lot of the difficulties we face could be met by realizing this possibility.

JENKINS: You might get a known-bacteriafree man, but I don't think you would get a virusfree man.

LIVINGSTON: Well, all right. Let the viruses go. We talk about germfree animals that carry viruses; that is a separate problem.

JENKINS: But there is a big problem. If you make a man bacteriafree, maybe you are going to run into real problems about fungi, viruses, and other things.

POLLARD: And not only that. Should he get exposed to another planet, he is hypersusceptible.

K. SCHWARZ: A bacteriafree animal is not a normal animal. You certainly would not have a normal man, for a number of reasons.

CALLOWAY: I was just thinking about the size of the appendix.

POLLARD: We established a new colony of germfree rabbits. One of the major problems of establishing this colony was a large cecum, to the extent that we were never able to establish a germfree rabbit until we just went in, opened him up, and cut off the cecum—the appendix, rather—and we have a colony going now.

But if you should envision a germfree man, you would have so many problems involved in stabilizing him, and especially in the gastrointestinal tract—

GUSTAFSSON: I am trying to get the floor to put things straight.

I was not suggesting that we are going to do it now, because, as Dr. Pollard said, we do not know all the germfree characteristics yet. I demonstrated some here yesterday, but there are about twenty of them and more to come.

Now, as we go on, however, we find that some of these characteristics are not harmful. Dr. Pollard mentioned the cecum enlargement, but that might be licked in another way, not by adding the living organisms, but the substances which are necessary for regulating this.

FREMONT-SMITH: Such as fibers, as you spoke of yesterday?

GUSTAFSSON: Such as the active amines, or whatever it is that creates the right tonus in the wall that is needed.

But I put forward this suggestion only to try to demonstrate to you that the germfree situation is a very well-defined and steady state as far as certain parameters are concerned, but that until we have found which are the germfree characteristics and how we are going to compensate for them, it is not a safe procedure to put a germfree man in space. I must underline that very strongly.

I would like to go on from there and tell that in 1956 there were only three laboratories in the whole world working with germfree animals. Now there are about thirty that I know of, and now you can buy germfree animals from the breeders, which shows a very definite exponential curve in activity.

Therefore, even if there are some germfree characteristics which are looking bad to us—the enlarged cecum, for example—in my opinion all these things will be licked sooner or later, and we will be able to compensate them not necessarily with microorganisms.

So if you want to, then, for any reason send a very well-defined man or animal, it would be the thing to do.

On reentry to the earth, there would be no problem, because, as I said, you can very easily give the total, balanced flora to the man immediately, and he would be in the same position as those animals which we are taking out from these isolators, which are not getting sick at all when we feed them the feces from normal animals.

POLLARD: Excepting guinea pigs. Guinea pigs die.

FREMONT-SMITH: If reinfected?

POLLARD: Yes, if they are taken out of germfree into a conventional environment, they die.

GUSTAFSSON: But you have not fed them with intestinal contents yet. You have to do that, because rats also die if you take them out.

POLLARD: Well, our rats survive very nicely, but our guinea pigs are very, very susceptible.

GUSTAFSSON: But you can condition that very easily. I can take out rats which are surviving, all of them, if I move them into an animal room, but they do not survive if I move them to my own office, so this can be conditioned all the way along, but you can always protect them by feeding them feces from normal animals.

MOSSEL: What do your guinea pigs die from when you expose them without intestinal implantation?

POLLARD: They die of almost anything that is in the environment; no specific organisms.

FREMONT-SMITH: But they die of some infection?

POLLARD: They die of some infection, yes.

MOSSEL: Whatever they may encounter, then; or, in other words, lack of sterility.

GUSTAFSSON: I have seen a septicemia with *Bacillus subtilis* in a mono-infected germfree rat.

BROWN: Yeast?

GUSTAFSSON: I have not seen that, but I would not say it would be impossible.

POLLARD: We contaminate our germfree rats with *Saccharomyces* as part of the defined flora and they seem to get along all right.

D. SCHWARZ: Do they get along better, for some reason?

POLLARD: No, we are just giving them a defined flora to provide us with a fairly decent control animal for the germfree counterparts, and we at least know what is in them. They get along fine.

POLLARD: There is another facet of this intestinal population that has to be taken into consideration, and that is the relationship of elements of that population to the immune status of the host.

Let us say an individual is exposed to a stressing situation. His resistance drops, and what we would ordinarily consider a sapropythic organism would then become pathogenic. This is again why I feel that defined flora must be considered seriously.

GUSTAFSSON: Here I can add that we have had a known mixture of six bacteria in an isolator with rats going on for one year without losing any of the contaminants. They are endosymbiotic bacteria and are behaving the same way now as they did when we started. So far it has been a very steady system.

K. SCHWARZ: May I say to that, though, that we are probably far away from really knowing all the microorganisms which are essential, so to speak.

GUSTAFSSON: Yes

FREMONT-SMITH: It seems to me that it would have been very interesting to have had a virologist here, because we have acted as if it did not matter what viruses there were. We know they are present in the germfree animals, and we know they are present in human beings.

POLLARD: They are not present in all germfree animals.

We have found thus far two viruses in germfree mice. We have found all mice infected with leukemia virus, and this is transmitted vertically, either transplacentally or through the ovum. They are born with it. We have found virus particles by electron microscopy in their thymuses at birth.

We have also found B particles in mammary carcinomas of germfree mice.

We have not been able to induce leukemia in germfree rats by irradiation. We have looked very extensively in target organs of rats for evidence of viruslike particles, and thus far we have found none.

There are certain target organs in animals that are very sensitive to exogenous agents—the lymph nodes, for instance—and in rats they are uniformly negative for the so-called germinal zones. You can add very minute amounts of antigens, for example, and within seven days you would find evidence of a response on the part of the host.

This is part of the answer. If these animals are born with an agent, they manifest what is known as immunologic tolerance, in which case they show neither disease nor antibodies. This is presently what we are working on, to see if we can analyze histologically and serologically the mechanism of immunologic tolerance in these animals, so that possibly we might be able to unmask more of the microbial agents in such animals.

But so far the rats are virusfree; the mice are not.

FREMONT-SMITH: Well, now, as far as the human problem in space, it seems to me still the question—and especially in the mixed infected food material—that we have to consider the possible impact of virus.

POLLARD: Most people are infected with herpes virus, and this is to some extent attuned to the immunologic status of the host, because there are certain periods—for instance, during the menstrual period—when a clinical case of herpes will recur. With men there are other episodes of stress, such as exposure to common colds, which are manifested by a herpes lesion.

I do not know how we can eliminate herpes from individuals. It can be a very severe disease, and can cause encephalitis and blindness. I do not think we should overlook the possibilities of latent or occult virus infections as possibly being manifested in the course of exposure to stressing environments.

FREMONT-SMITH: In three years in space.

POLLARD: Yes.

MUNRO: With regard to the normal flora of the intestinal tract, or the standard flora, is it possible to recommend a flora which will have minimal gas formation, and therefore give rise to less distention at reduced pressures? Would this be a point in establishing a standard flora?

MAYER: I did not think there was any plan to send people on very long missions on abnormal atmospheres. In other words, the type of atmosphere that exists now is a temporary expedient until the walls can become thicker, is it not?

ARNOLDI: The walls of the vehicle? Yes.

GUSTAFSSON: But is it not so, if I may ask, that even under the conditions prevailing on these flights—has there been any distress from gas formation, distention, and so forth? Or have you tested this on the ground in reduced pressure systems?

What is the knowledge of these symptoms at present in the studies you have already made?

CALLOWAY: In simulator studies they complain with some regularity. I have not seen any reports from astronauts in actual flights.

GUSTAFSSON: Because I would think that those are symptoms to be experienced only during change in conditions like pressure. The reduced pressure after take off would not cause any trouble, when it has stabilized itself.

REYNOLDS: Before flight they are denitrogenated, which would help.

POLLARD: Dr. Fenn, there is one matter which I had intended to bring in regarding the intestinal flora. Our radiation biologist has been examining germfree mice for response to x-ray exposure, and he has monocontaminated them with specific organisms. Certain of them, with *Clostridium difficule,* show increased resistance to the damaging effects of irradiation to the extent of 100 roentgens. Others, of course, show a hypersusceptibility or increased sensitivity to x ray.

Here again the intestinal flora may be of some significance, in so far as the carrier is concerned. There is a modifying effect of the intestinal flora on response to the environment.

FENN: I am impressed how long it has taken to design man so that he can tolerate the conditions that we have on the earth, and it is not remarkable that it takes more than a few years to fix conditions so that he can survive in a space capsule.

I wonder how we ever survive as it is, with all the hazards presented to us that might happen to us with very slight changes. We are really lucky to be alive, every one of us, with all these threats on every side: a slight change in the intestinal flora or some latent virus, or a trace mineral deficiency.

FREMONT-SMITH: Some of us are not.

FENN: Some of us are not, but it has taken many years to weed out the unfit.

MUNRO: One thing that is quite clear is that there is a tremendous interaction, so that you cannot move in one direction without also making an adjustment in the other.

You cannot think about intestinal populations without bringing in at the same time the question of what type of diet, whether this is *Chlorella* or some other material, and I feel that the value of this meeting rests in giving us these additional perspectives to warn us—not that they solve any problems, because they raise a very large number of them.

FREMONT-SMITH: Will any of you who have suggestions as to how we could run this kind of a conference more effectively please drop us a line? We would welcome it. This is still an experiment in progress, and we need your help. Thank you very much.

FENN: I might make some wise comment about what this Conference has accomplished, but I shall not try to do that, except on an individual basis. I shall simply say that I have learned a lot.

I thank you all very much for coming, and I would like to thank The New York Academy of Sciences, Dr. Frank Fremont-Smith, Mrs. Purcell, and Miss Gordon, for all their help and everything they have done for us.

REFERENCES

1. Schwarz, K. 1964. Conference on Nutrition in Space and Related Waste Problems. Univ. of South Florida, Tampa, Fla., April 27–30, NASA Report SP-70.
2. Miller, W. 1964. Looking for the General. McGraw-Hill Book Co., Inc. New York.
3. Winitz, M., Graff, J., Gallagher, N., Narkin, A. & Seedman, D. A. 1965. Evaluation of chemical diets as nutrition for man-in-space. Nature **205:** 741–743.
4. Winitz, M., Graff, J. & Seedman, D. A. 1964. Arch. Biochem. Biophys. **108:** 576.
5. Anonymous. 1965. The use of chemically defined diets in metabolic studies in man. Nutrition Rev. **23:** 231.
6. Macdonald, I. & Braithwaite, D. M. 1964. Clin. Sci. 27: 23; Macdonald, I., Ed. 1967. Symposium on Dietary Carbohydrates in Man. Am. J. Clin. Nutrition **20**(2): 65–208.
7. FAO Committee. 1957. Protein Requirements. FAO Nutritional Studies No. 16. Food and Agricultural Organization. Rome, Italy.
8. Joint FAO/WHO Expert Group. 1965. Protein Requirements. WHO Tech. Rept. Series No. 301. World Health Organization. Geneva, Switzerland.
9. Martin, C. J. & Robison, R. 1922. The minimum nitrogen expenditure of man and the biological value of various proteins for human nutrition. Biochem. J. **16:** 406–447.
10. Bricker, M. L., Shiveley, R. F., Smith, J. M., Mitchell, H. H. & Hamilton, T. S. 1949. The protein requirements of college women on high cereal diets with observation on the adequacy of short balance periods. J. Nutrition **37:** 163–183.
11. Munro, H. N. 1964. *In* Munro, H. N. & Allison, J. B., Eds. Mammalian Protein Metabolism, Vol. I, Chap. 10. Academic Press, New York.
12. Calloway, D. H. & Margen, S. 1967. Fed. Proc. **26:** 629.
13. Sirbu, E. R., Margen, S. & Calloway, D. H. 1967. Fed. Proc. **26:** 629.
14. Kies, C., Williams, E. & Fox, H. M. 1965. Effect of "non-specific" nitrogen intake on adequacy of cereal proteins for nitrogen retention in human adults. J. Nutrition **86:** 357–361.
15. Reissmann, K. R. 1964. Protein metabolism and erythropoiesis. I. The anemia of protein deprivation. Blood **23:** 137–145.
16. Consolazio, C. F., Nelson, R. A., Natoush, L. O., Harding, R. S. & Canham, J. E. 1963. Nitrogen excretion in sweat and its relation to nitrogen balance requirements. J. Nutrition **79:** 399–406.
17. Mitchell, H. H. & Hamilton, T. S. 1949. The dermal excretion under controlled environmental conditions of nitrogen and minerals in human subjects, with particular reference to calcium and iron. J. Biol. Chem. **178:** 345–361.
18. Silwer, H. 1937. Studien über die N-Ausscheidung im Harn bei Einschränkung des Kohlenhydratgehaltes der Nahrung ohne wesentliche Veränderung des Energiegehaltes derselben. Acta Med. Scand. Suppl. **79:** 1–271.
19. McClellan, W. S. & DuBois, E. F. 1930. Clinical calorimetry. XLV. Prolonged meat diets with a study of kidney function and ketosis. J. Biol. Chem. **87:** 651–668.

20. Stefansson, V. 1956. The Fat of the Land. The Macmillan Co. New York.
21. Shaffer, P. A. 1922. J. Biol. Chem. **50**: 26.
22. Renner, R. & Elcombe, A. L. 1964. J. Nutrition **84**: 327.
23. Rose, W. C., Coon, M. J. & Lambert, G. F. 1954. The amino acid requirements of man. VI. The rate of the caloric intake. J. Biol. Chem. **210**: 331.
24. Geiger, E. & Nimni, M. 1958. Effect of dietary carbohydrate and fat on utilization of essential amino acids in rats. Fed. Proc. **17**: 476.
25. Schwarz, K., Smith, J. C. & Oda, T. A. 1966. Fed. Proc. **25**: 542.
26. Smith, J. C. & Schwartz, K. 1966. Fed. Proc. **25**: 432.
27. Schwarz, K. & Mertz, W. 1959. Arch. Biochem. Biophys. **85**: 292.
28. Schwarz, K. & Mertz, W. 1961. Fed. Proc. **20**: Suppl. 10, 11.
29. Schwarz, K. & Foltz, C. M. 1957. J. Am. Chem. Soc. **79**: 3292.
30. Schwarz, K. & Mertz, W. 1957. Arch. Biochem. Biophys. **72**: 515.
31. Chatin, A. 1850–1854. Compt. Rend. Acad. Sci. 30–39.
32. Hart, E. B., Steenbock, H., Waddell, J. & Elvehjem, C. A. 1928. J. Biol. Chem. **77**: 797.
33. Kemmerer, A. R. & Todd, W. R. 1931. J. Biol. Chem. **94**: 317.
34. Todd, W. R., Elvehjem, C. A. & Hart, E. B. 1934. Am. J. Physiol. **107**: 146.
35. Underwood, E. J. & Filmer, J. F. 1935. Austral. Vet. J. **11**: 84.
36. Marston, H. R. 1935. J. Council Sci. Ind. Res. **8**: 111.
37. Lines, E. W. 1935. J. Council Sci. Ind. Res. **8**: 117.
38. de Renzo, E. C., Kaleita, E., Heytler, P., Oleson, J. J., Hutchings, B. L. & Williams, J. H. 1953. J. Am. Chem. Soc. **75**: 753.
39. Richert, D. A. & Westerfeld, W. W. 1953. J. Biol. Chem. **203**: 915.
40. Mertz, W. & Schwarz, K. 1959. Am. J. Phys. **196**: 614.
41. Schroeder, H. A. 1966. J. Nutrition **88**: 439.
42. Glinsmann, W. & Mertz, W. 1966. Abstracts papers VIIth Internl. Congr. Nutrition, Hamburg, Aug. 3–10, p. 264.
43. Mertz, W., Roginski, E. E. & Schwarz, K. 1963. J. Biol. Chem. **238**: 868.
44. Christian, G. D., Knoblock, E. C., Purdy, W. C. & Mertz, W. 1963. Biochem. Biophys. Acta **66**: 420.
45. Glinsmann, W., Feldman, F. J. & Mertz, W. 1966. Science **152**: 1243.
46. Feldman, F. J. & Purdy, W. C. 1965. Anal. Chem. Acta **33**: 273.
47. Hopkins, Jr., L. L. & Schwarz, W. 1964. Biochem. Biophys. Acta **90**: 484.
48. Lewis, J. & Wilkins, R. G. 1960. Modern Coordination Chemistry. Interscience Publishers, Inc. New York.
49. Underwood, E. J. 1962. Trace Elements in Human and Animal Nutrition. Academic Press. New York & London.
50. Magee, A. C. & Matrone, G. 1960. J. Nutrition **72**: 233.
51. Bosshardt, D. K., Huff, J. W. & Barnes, R. H. 1956. Proc. Soc. Exptl. Biol. Med. **92**: 219.
52. Kar, A. B., Das, R. T. & Mukerji, B. 1960. Proc. Natl. Inst. Sci. (India) **26B**: 40.
53. Mason, K. E. & Young, J. O. 1965. Anatomical Record **151**: 382.
54. Symposium on Interaction of Mineral Elements in Nutrition and Metabolism. 1960. Fed. Proc. **19**: 635.
55. Schwarz, K. & Foltz, C. M. 1958. J. Biol. Chem. **233**: 245.
56. Schwarz, K. 1948. Z. Physiol. Chem. **283**: 186.

57. (Schwarz: missing).
58. Bosshardt, D. K., Huff, J. W. & Barnes, R. H. 1956. Effect of bromine on chick growth. Proc. Soc. Exptl. Biol. Med. **92:** 219–221.
59. Huff, J. W., Bosshardt, D. K., Miller, O. P. & Barnes, R. H. 1956. A nutritional requirement for bromine. Proc. Soc. Exptl. Biol. Med. **92:** 216–219.
60. McClendon, J. F. & Gershon-Cohen, J. 1953. Trace element deficiencies: Water culture crops designed to study deficiencies in animals. J. Agr. Food Chem. **1:** 464–466.
61. Maurer, R. L. & Day, H. G. 1957. The non-essentiality of fluorine. J. Nutrition **62:** 561–573.
62. McClendon, J. F. & Gershon-Cohen, J. 1958. Fluorine and dental caries. J. Albert Einstein Med. Center : 153–154.
63. Orland, F. J., Blayney, J. P., Harrison, R. W., Reyniers, J. A., Trexler, P. C., Wagner, M., Gordon, H. A. & Luckey, T. D. 1954. Use of germ-free animal technique in the study of experimental dental caries. I. Basic observations on rats reared free of all microorganisms. J. Dental Res. **33:** 147–174.
64. Wagner, M. & Orland, F. 1964. The possible influence of salivary antibody on experimental dental caries in gnotobiotic rats. Proc. Indiana Acad. Sci. **73:** 75.
65. Nachman, M. 1963. Learned aversion to the taste of lithium chloride and generalization to other salts. J. Comp. Physiol. Psychol. **56:** 343–349.
66. Wood, J. D. & Watson, W. J. 1963. Gamma-aminobutyric acid levels in the brain of rats exposed to oxygen at high pressures. Canad. J. Biochem. Physiol. **41:** 1907–1913.
67. Thomas, J. J., Neptune, E. M. & Sudduth, H. C. 1963. Toxic effects of oxygen at high pressures on the metabolism of D-glucose by dispersions of rat brain. Biochem. J. **88:** 31–45.
68. Michel, E. L., Langevin, R. W. & Gell, C. F. 1960. Effect of continuous human exposure to oxygen tension of 418 mm Hg for 168 hours. Aerospace Med. **31:** 138–144.
69. Harper, J. C. & Tappel, A. L. 1957. Freeze-drying of food products. Adv. Food Res. **7:** 172–232.
70. Brobeck, J. R. 1964. Food requirements in space. *In* Hardy, J. D., Ed. Physiological Problems in Space Exploration. 134–151. Charles C Thomas. Springfield, Ill.
71. Cuthbertson, D. P. & Munro, H. N. 1939. The relationship of carbohydrate metabolism to protein metabolism. I. The roles of total dietary carbohydrate and of surfeit carbohydrate in protein metabolism. Biochem. J. **33:** 128–139.
72. Tepperman, J., Brobeck, J. R. & Long, C. N. H. 1943. Yale J. Biol. Med. **15:** 875.
73. Van Putten, L. M., Van Bekkum, D. W. & Querido, A. 1955. Influence of hypothalamic lesions producing hyperphagia and of feeding regimens on carcass composition of the rat. Metabolism **4:** 68–73.
74. Cohn, C. & Joseph, D. 1955. Effect of food administration on weight gains and body composition of normal and adrenalectomized rats. Am. J. Physiol. **180:** 503–557.
75. Cohn, C. & Joseph, D. 1959. Changes in body composition attendant on force feeding. Am. J. Physiol. **196:** 965–968.

76. HOLLIFIELD, G. & PARSEN, W. 1962. Metabolic adaptations to "Stuff and Starve" feeding program. II. Obesity and the persistence of adaptive changes in adipose tissue and liver occurring in rats limited to a short daily feeding period. J. Clin. Invest. **41**: 251–253.
77. TEPPERMAN, J., BROBECK, J. R. & LONG, C. N. H. 1943. The effects of hypothalamic hyperphagia and of alterations in feeding habits on the metabolism of the albino rat. Yale J. Biol. Med. **15**: 855–874.
78. FALRY, P., FODOR, J., HEJL, Z., BRAUN, T. & ZVOLANKOVA, K. 1964. The frequency of meals, its relation to overweight, hypercholesteraemia and decreases in glucose tolerance. Lancet **2**: 614–615.
79. GIVENUP, G., BRYON, R. C., ROUSH, W., KURGER, F. & HAMWI, G. J. 1963. The effect of nibbling versus gorging on glucose tolerance. Lancet **2**: 165–167.
80. WU, H. & WU, D. Y. 1950. Influence of feeding schedule on nitrogen utilization and excretion. Proc. Soc. Exptl. Biol. Med. **74**: 78–81.
81. LEVERTON, R. M. & GRAM, M. R. 1949. Nitrogen excretion of women related to the distribution of animal protein in daily meals. J. Nutrition **39**: 57–65.
82. COHN, C. & JOSEPH, D. 1960. Effects on metabolism produced by the rate of ingestion of the diet: "Meal eating" versus "Nibbling." Am. J. Clin. Nutrition **8**: 682.
83. RICHTER, C. P. 1922. A behavioristic study of the activity of the rat. Comp. Psychol. Monogr. **1**: 1–55.
84. HAMMEL, H. T., ELSNER, R. W., LE MESSURIES, D. H. ANDERSON, H. T. & MILAN, F. A. 1959. Thermal and metabolic responses of the Australian aborigine exposed to moderate cold in summer. J. Appl. Physiol. **14**: 605–615.
85. ARBIT, J., SUNDERLAND, J. E. & COHEN, J. Appraisal of Psychomotor Performance in Man and Dogs. Dept. of Army contract No. DA–19–129–QM–1539, Northwestern University, Evanston, Illinois.
86. SHERRINGTON, C. A. 1900. The spinal cord. *In* Schäfer, E. A., Ed. Textbook of Physiology. Vol. 2. Young J. Pentland. Edinburgh.
87. SHELDON, W. H., STEVENS, S. S. & TUCKER, W. B. 1940. The Varieties of Human Physique. Harper & Bros. New York.
88. HALBERG, F. 1964. Physiologic rhythms. *In* Hardy, J. D., Ed. Physiological Problems in Space Exploration. 298–322. Charles C Thomas. Springfield, Ill.
89. EPSTEIN, A. N. & TEITELBAUM, P. 1962. Regulation of food intake in the absence of taste, smell and other oropharyngeal sensations. J. Comp. Physiol. Psychol. **55**: 753–759.
90. WEIJERS, H. A. & VAN DE KRAMER, J. H. 1965. Alterations of intestinal bacterial flora as a cause of diarrhea. Nutr. Abstr. Rev. **35**: 591–604.
91. HOROWITZ, D., LOVENBERG, W., ENGELMAN, K. & SJOERDSMA, A. 1964. Mono-amino-oxidase inhibitors, tyramine, and cheese. J. Am. Med. Assoc. **188**: 1108 1110.
92. BORGSTRÖM, B., DAHLQVIST, A., LUNDH, G., & SJÖVALL, J. 1957. Studies of digestion and absorption in the human. J. Clin. Invest. **36**: 1521.
93. CALLOWAY, D. H., COLASITO, D. J. & MATHEWS, R. D. 1966. Nature (London) **212**: 1238.
94. CALLOWAY, D. H. & MURPHY, E. L. 1967. Ann. N.Y. Acad. Sci. (in press).
95. ZOBELL, C. E. & OPPENHEIMER, C. H. 1950. Some effects of hydrostatic pressure on the multiplication and morphology of marine bacteria. J. Bacteriol. **60**: 771–781.

96. Gall, L. S. 1966. Study of the normal fecal bacterial flora of man. NASA Contractor Rept. CR-467, p. 43.
97. Schaedler, R. W., Dubos, R., & Costello, R. 1965. Association of germ-free mice with bacteria isolated from normal mice. J. Exp. Med. **122:** 77.
98. Lev, M., Alexander, R. H., & Levenson, S. M. 1966. Stability of the Lactobacillus population in feces and stomach contents of rats prevented from coprophagy. J. Bacteriol. **92:** 13.
99. Teah, B. A. 1885–1963. Bibliography of Germfree Research. Lobund Laboratory, University of Notre Dame. Notre Dame, Ind. 1964. Suppl. 1965.
100. Moyer, J. E. 1964. Microbiological problems of sealed cabin environments. Dev. Ind. Microbiol. **5:** 216–223.
101. Major, C. J. 1966. Gaseous diffusion cells. *In* Kammermeyer, K., Ed. Atmosphere in Space Cabins and Closed Environments. Appleton-Century-Crofts. New York.
102. Arnoldi, W. E. 1966. An electrolytic process for carbon dioxide separation and oxygen reclamation. *In* Kammermeyer, K., Ed. Atmosphere in Space Cabins and Closed Environments. Appleton-Century-Crofts. New York.
103. Miller, R. L. & Ward, C. H. 1966. Algal bioregenerative systems. *In* Kammermeyer, K., Ed. Atmosphere in Space Cabins and Closed Environments. Appleton-Century-Crofts. New York.
104. Krauss, R. W. 1962. Mass culture of algae for food and other organic compounds. Am. J. Bot. **49:** 425–435.
105. Krauss, R. W. & Osretkar, A. 1961. Minimum and maximum tolerance of algae to temperature and light intensity. *In* Campbell, P. A., Ed. The Medical and Biological Aspects of the Energetics of Space. 253–273. Columbia Univ. Press. New York.
106. Engel, R. W. 1954. Mineral and vitamin requirements of long flights. *In* Conference on Nutrition in Space and Related Waste Problems. 147–153. Scientific and Technical Information Div. NASA. Washington, D.C.
107. Sargent, II, F. & Johnson, R. E. 1958. The physiological basis for various constituents in survival rations. IV. An integrative study of the all-purpose survival ration for temperate, cold and hot weather. WADC Tech. Rept. 53–484. Wright-Patterson Air Force Base, Ohio.
108. Becker, R. O., Bassett, C. A. & Bachman, C. H. 1964. Bioelectrical factors controlling bone structure. *In* Frost, Ed. Bone Biodynamics. Little, Brown & Co., Inc. New York.

INDEX

Acceptability
- of biomasses as food, 199-203, 219
- of food, 222-223

Acids, in feces of breastfed and artificially fed, 128, 130, 131
Aging, process of, 77-78
Algae
- bioregeneration with, 190-195
- in bioregenerative systems, 180-188
- contamination of, in cultures, 214-216
- cultured in different atmospheres, 219-220
- and goldfish in closed ecology, 74
- lyphilization of, 214
- nutritive value of, 188
- recyclostat to produce, 191-192
- requirements of, for space missions, 189
- use of, for animal and human food, 188-195

Algal cultures
- on other planets, 222
- sterile versus contaminated, 217-219

Algal regenerative systems, illumination engineering for, 181-184
Algal system, 160
- regenerative, for space flight, 181-188
- weight of, 187-188

Algalburgers, 185
Alpha-tocopherol, optimum amounts of, 84-85
Amines
- biogenic, 133
- toxicity from, 135

Amino acid diet, composition of, 67
Ammonia, lack of, in gases evolved during anaerobic fermentation in *vitro,* 138
Animals
- germfree characteristics in normal, 154
- sterilization of, for "germfreeing," 157-158

Antioxidants
- in closed ecology, 90
- and free radical scavengers, 84
- need for, in space travel, 80
- and oxidation in space flight, 74-88 *passim*
- synthetic, 85

Apollo, as Phase II mission, 163
Appetite, satiety, food acceptance and, 92-118
Astronauts
- cardiovascular reflexes in, 88
- causes of death among, 208-209
- decalcification in, 88
- diet conditioning of, 115, 117, 118
- gas in stomach of, 137
- germfree, 223-231 *passim*
- intestinal flora in, 119
- maintenance of biological cycles in, 108-109
- minimal intestinal flora for, 157
- nutritional requirements of, 44-47
- oxygen poisoning in, 82-83
- screening of, 91
- sleep-wakefulness cycle in, 108
- toxicity of, to organisms, 221
- water balance in, 88

Atmosphere regeneration, chemical systems of, 161-176 *passim*
Australian Aborigine, food patterns in, 101
Autooxidation, polyunsaturated fatty acids and, 86, 87

Bacteria
- cooperation between insects and, 120-121
- in coprophagic rats, 140, 141
- enteric, in man, 125-127
- hydrocarbons produced by, vary with pressure, 137
- in ileocecal area, 129-130
- intestinal
  - data on formation of aliphatic acids by, 127
  - general metabolic activity of, 125, 126
  - sites of, in man, 121-127
- in large intestine, 139
- in lumen, 139, 140
- in mouth and intestine, 122
- in mucosa, 139-140
- in noncoprophagic rats, 140, 141
- oceanic marine, variations of, in chain length of hydrocarbons, 137
- as potential for food, 197, 198

Bacteria—Continued
  shift in predominant anaerobic, in space-type diet, 156
  in stomach and small intestine, 139
  strains of, in intestinal contents, 122-123
Bacteriodes spp., form propionic acid, 125
Bile acids, delayed turnover of, in germfree rat, 43
Biological cycles, maintenance of, 108-114
Biomasses, acceptability of, as food, 199-203, 219
Bioregeneration, with algae, 190-195
Bioregenerative system, 160, 179-188 *passim*
  activation time for, 179-180
  stability of, 213-223
  temperature for, 179
Birds, function of obesity in migrating, 100-101
Blood cholesterol, feeding pattern and, 99
Bone, fluorides and formation of, 70
Bone marrow, sensitivity of, to protein in diet, 39
Bromide, in nutrition, 70
Browning, destroys histidine and lysine, 79

CO_2

  control of, in space flight, 166-176
  electrolytic cell schematic diagram of, 172, 173
  separation
    ion exchange resin concept for, 170-171
    regenerable solid adsorbent system for, 167-168
    for semipermeable membrane concept, 169-170
Caloric balances, in space capsule, 25
Calorie intakes
  adaptation to, 212
  survival time and, 209-210
  consumption of, 99
  expenditure of, in space flight, 207-210
  and utilization of dietary protein, 48
Cannibalism, in rats and mice, 144-145
Carbohydrates
  as essential in diet, 51
  serum cholesterol, diets, and 31-32
Carbon dioxide control system, principles of, 166-167
Cardiovascular reflexes, in astronauts, 88-90
Cellular damage, free radicals and peroxides in *in vivo,* 75, 76
Chemical systems, of atmospheric regenerations, 161-176 *passim*
Chlorella, species of, for bioregeneration, 190-191
Chloretta sorokiniana, yield of, in long-term
  Recyclostat experiments, 194-195, 196
Chlorella vannielli, yield of, in long-term Recyclostat experiments, 193-195
Cholic acid, elimination of, in conventional and germfree rats, 152, 153
Chromium
  abundance of effective levels of, 57
  action of, 58
  binding of, 58
  as bioelement, 55, 56-61
  as cofactor of insulin, 58
  correlation between diabetes and, 57
  effect of highly specific, 58
  glucose tolerance factor-potency complexes of, 57
  physiological role of, 56
  transported by transferrin, 58
Circadian cycles, 109, 110, 111, 113
Closed ecology, 71-74, 160, 163
  antioxidants in, 90
  goldfish and algae in, 74
  for space flights, 116
Clostridia
  in methane-producing subjects, 136
  as pathogenic, 127
Colitis nervosa, pattern in, 136
Contamination, among germfree rats, 145-146
Convulsions, oxygen pressure and, 83
Cooking, and food habits, 96
Coprophagy, in rat, 43, 140, 141
Coronary catastrophe, and space travel, 32

Cycle
body temperature, 111, 118
biological, 108-114
circadian, 109, 110, 111, 113
diurnal, 108, 110, 111
potassium, 111
sleep, 111
sleep-wakefulness, 108
in space flight, 112, 113
watch, 112-113
Cysteamine, protective action against radiation, 79

Decalcification, in astronauts, 88
Defecation, in space flight, 21
Dehydration
and food consumption, 114
and thirst, 21
voluntary, 25
Dental caries, in rat, 71
Desquamation, loss by, from epidermis, 41, 42
Diabetes
correlation between chromium and, 57-58
impaired glucose tolerance and, 57
Diarrhea
bacteriology and biochemistry of, 131-136
fermentative, 131, 132
proteolytic, 133, 135
putrefactive, 132-133, 134
Diet
acceptance of bland, 117
algal, 223
amino acid, 50, 51
application of defined, to space flight, 29-31
carbohydrates and serum cholesterol, 31-32
chemically defined, and space flight, 29-21
composition of amino acid, 67
and composition of food, 98
composition of semisynthetic, for germfree rats, 143-146
desiccated thyroid in, 70
effect of, on efficiency, 117
energy-yielding constituents of, 29
fluoride-free, 71
formula, 30, 31, 117, 199, 200-201, 211, 212, 216, 222
interaction of, and flora in man, 210-211
for mice, 224
high-carbohydrate, 50
high-fat, and ketosis, 49
infection and low-protein, 53
loss of nitrogen and carbohydrate-free, 48
and mental apathy, 52
natural, 222
urinary secretion of ntrogen, in protein-free, 33-34
protein-fat, 48-49
protein loss on protein-free, 33-34
relation of, and intestinal flora, 140
semisynthetic, 210
shift in predominant anaerobic bacteria in space-type, 156
soft, 30
and increase in fecal output, 31
synthetic, 31-32
involving amino acid mixtures, 50, 51
tradition of high protein, 50
and waste disposal, 116, 118
Diurnal cycles, 108, 110, 111
maintenance of, 108, 110, 111
Dog, alertness after feeding in, 105
Drift
in body temperature cycles, 108
of intestinal flora, 119
Dysbacteriosis
defined, 124
fermentative, 134
pattern in putrefactive, 136
proteolytic, 137

E. coli, in stools of man, 123, 125
Eating, and neuropsychiatric responsiveness, 103-108
Ecology, recycling system in closed, 71-74
Endosymbionts, culture of, 156
Endosymbiosis, 119, 120, 121, 152, 154
Energy, expenditure of, and food intake, 97-98
Enterocolitis, 129

Environment, control of, in Mercury, Gemini, and Apollo programs, 160
Equilibrium-states and amino acid nutrition, 54
Eubacteriosis
  defined, 124
  in adults, 124-125

Factor G, 91
Fasting
  in rats, 115
  versus starving, 106
Fats, "overheated," 87
Feces, analysis of, after diet trials, 30-31
Feeding
  and composition of diet, 98
  frequency of, 97-103
    in rats, 100
  habits, 99-100
  and nitrogen balance studies, 97
  patterns of, 108-113
    and blood cholesterol, 99
  and reward, 104
  synthetic mixtured, 50
Flatus, nitrogen in, 138, 139
Flora
  bacterial, and man on space flight, 224
  bile acid metabolism of intestinal, 154
  defined, in germfree animals, 224
  interaction of formula diet and, in man, 210-211
  interaction of, and man, 187, 198
  intestinal
    in astronauts, 156
    in germfree animals, 119
    and germfree life, 119-159
    in healthy children and adults, 123-124
    Lactobacilli in, 122
    in man, and space flights, 123-136
    minimal, for astronaut, 157
    minimal, for developing germfree characteristics, 119, 157
    in monogastric animals, 119
  reestablishment of, 225
  reinoculation of man with, 225-226
  relation of diet and intestinal, 140
  standardization of intestinal, in man, 211
Fluoride
  effect of, in osteoporosis, 70
  and formation of bone, 70
Food
  acceptability of, 222-223
  appetite, satiety, and acceptance of, 92-118
  chemical synthesis of, for space flight, 176-179
  consumption of, and dehydration, 114
  control of intake of, by nervous system, 92
  deprivation, and acceptance of, 95
  and emotional values, 103-105
  forms of, for space flight, 210-213
  heat treatment of, 87
  intake of, and energy expenditure, 97-98
  need for compressed, 24
  packaging of, 24
  patterns of, in Australian Aborigine, 101
  and personality traits, 107-108
  preference of, 92, 93-94
  processing of, 201-202, 203
    and weight per man, 205
  storage versus generation of, 115-116
  and stress, 106-107
  synthesized, of life in space, 28-29
  technology of, for man in space, 202-203
  temperature, and intake of, 101
  training in acceptance of, 94, 96
  as tranquilizer, 105
  use of dehydrated, 19
  variety of, versus formula diets, 22-27
  weight of, for space flight, 116
Food habits
  changes in, 95-96
  and cooking technology, 96
  experience, training, and, 93-96
Food supplies of astronauts, 21-22
Formula diets, variety of food versus, 22
Fuel cell
  usefulness of, 20
  workings of, 29

Gases
  examination of flatus and respiratory, 137, 138-139

Gases—Continued
production of, in relation to flatulence, 136
Gemini series, 17-18
Genetic drift, and metabolism, 213-214
Germfree animals, 226, 227, 229, 230
defined flora in, 224
rearing of, 141
Germfree capsule, 226
Germfree rabbits, 226
Germfree research, 140-159
Glucose tolerance factor (GTF), 56-59
Gold, biological effect of, 69-70
Goldfish, and algae in closed ecology, 74
Gravity, effect on metabolism, 212-213

Heat stress
and loss of nitrogen, 40
and adrenocortical stimulation, 40
Heat treatment, of food, 87
Hibernation
and loss of nitrogen, 44
and reduction of caloric needs, 44
Histidine, browning destroys, 79
Human being, problem of maintaining, during space flight and in outer space, 15, 16
Hunger
effect on nervous system, 105
and hydration, 114
and performance, 103-106
and satiety, 97
Hydration, and hunger, 114
Hydrocarbons, produced by bacteria vary with pressure, 137
Hydrogen, production of, in breath, 136
Hydrogenomonas
bioregenerative system, 203
toxicity of, 217
Hydrogenomonas eutropha, bacterial system, 195-198
Hydrogenomonas system, 160
Hydrolysis, and olation, 60
Hysterectomy, effect on enteric seeds, 130

Implantation therapy, 225
Incubator system for trace-element controlled environment, 66
Infection, and low-protein diet, 53
Ion exchange resin concept for CO_2 separation, 170-171
Insects, cooperation between bacteria and, 120-121
Insulin, chromium as cofactor of, 58
Isolators
plastic, for germfree research, 141-143
stainless steel, for germfree research, 141-143

K ration, 96
Ketosis, and high-fat diet, 49

Lactobacilli
fecal counts of, in rats and vitamin-K-deficient diet, 141
in intestinal flow, 122
in walls of stomach of mice, 140
Leak rate, in Mercury capsule, 160
Lesion, and emotional behavior in rats, 102-103
Lipids, thermal degradative changes in, 87
Lithium
relation to metabolic process, 73
toxic in rat, 73
to treat manic depressive psychosis, 73
Lithium compounds, in atmospheric control systems, 72
Lithium hydroxide
for Apollo mission, 163
for CO_2 control, 166-167
Loss, fecal, 41-42
Lumen, bacteria in, 139, 140
Lysine
browning destroys, 79
sensitivity to heat, 79

Macronutrients, 28-53, 207
Man
enteric bacteria in, 125-127
and flora bacterial on space flight, 224
germfree, as abnormal, 158
interaction of flora and, 187, 198
interaction of formula diet and flora in, 210-211
intestinal flora in, 121-127
and space flight, 123-136
protein requirements in, 32-40
reinoculation of, with flora, 225-226
standardization of intestinal flora in, 211
under germfree conditions, 158

Man-machine interrelationship, 14
Meals, frequency of, 97-113
Membrane packages, for multistage systems, 170
Mental apathy and diet, 52
Mercury capsule, leak rate in, 160
Mercury series, experience from, 17
Metal, 59
Methane
  production of
    in relation to flatulence, 136
    via lungs, 137
Methionine
  as liable amino acid, 79
  as protector against radiation, 79
  sensitivity to heat, 79
Mice, formula diet for, 224
Microflora, intestinal, and germfree life, 119-159
Micronutrients, 206
  relation to lengthy space missions, 54-91
Mucin, in feces and contents of large intestine of germfree rat, 151
Mucosa, bacteria in, 139, 140
Mycetomes, 120

Nervous system
  control of food intake by, 92
  effect of hunger on, 105
Neutron-activation analysis for determination of elements on moon, 64
Nitrogen
  balance of, in healthy young men, 38
  basal output of, in urine, 34, 35
  cutaneous loss of, 40-41
  depletion and repletion in diet trials, 30
  in flatus, 138, 139
  input and output of, in adult rat, 42-43
  loss of, 138n.
    basal, 37
    and carbohydrate-free diet, 48
    dermal and intestinal, 40-43
    and heatstress, 40
    and hibernation, 44
    sweat, 40-41
    and urea levels, 37
  measurement of
    loss from skin, 40-41
    output of urinary, fecal, and cutaneous, 37
  usefulness of labile, 36
Nitrogen balance studies and feeding, 97
Nonpathogenic agents, 127, 129
Nutrient requirements, for space flight, 206-210
Nutrition
  bromide in, 70
  international requirements of, 35, 36
  and quality attributes, 23-27
  selectivity and specificity of trace element requirements in, 39
  in space, and waste problems, 116, 118

Obesity, in migrating birds, 100-101
Oblation, and hydrolysis, 60
Odor, and taste, 114-115
Orbiting laboratories, 160
Osteoporosis, effect of fluoride in, 70
Overheating, in spacecraft, 89
Oxidation, and antioxidants, in space flight, 74-88
Oxygen
  maximum partial pressure, and survival, 85
  poisoning, 75, 81
  in astronauts, 82-83
Oxygen pressure, and convulsions, 83
Oxygen reclamation systems
  Bosch process, 171, 172, 176, 177
  fused lithium carbonate electrolysis, 171, 172-174, 175, 177
  Sabatier process, 171, 172, 176, 178
  solid electrolyte, 171, 173-175, 177-178
Oxygen tension, and decrease in radiation sensitivity, 84

Pathogenicity, of enteric organisms, 127-136
Performance, and hunger, 103-106
Peroxidation
  as deteriorative reaction, 77-79
  and food stability in space travel, 86-87
  of polyunsaturated lipids, 75
Peroxides, organic, as harmful, 77
Photosynthetic regeneration, 184
  stages of, 181
Polyunsaturated fatty acids, susceptible to autoxidation, 86, 87

Polyunsaturated lipids, nutritional requirement of, 80-81
Populations, nutritional requirements of, 46-47
Potassium cycle, 111
Protein
  calories and utilization of dietary, 48
  intake of, and injury and infection, 52-53
  loss of body, 53
  minimal daily requirement of, 35
  replacement of body, with dietary, 35
  requirements of
    in man, 32-40
    and optimum performances, 47-48
    range of, 43-44
    in strenuous work, 52
  sensitivity of bone marrow to, in diet, 39
  whole, in diet trials, 30
Protein reaction, peroxidizing-lipid, compared to protein radiation and age pigment, 77-79
Proteus, in stools of man, 123, 125
Protoplasm, rejection and use of, 221
Psychosis, lithium to treat, 73

Radiation
  damage from at cellular level, 77
  exposure to, on space flights, 75
  protection against, 77, 79, 85
  shielding from, 77
  from solar flares, 75
  sulfhydryl compounds as protectors from, 77
  in van Allen belt, 75
Radiation preservation, 202
Rats
  bacteria in coprophagic and noncoprophagic, 140, 141
  capacity for increase in protein content of liver cells, 36
  coprohagy in, 43
  delayed turnover of bile acids in germfree, 43
  dental caries in, 71
  fasting in, 115
  fecal counts of *Lactobacilli* in, on vitamin-K-deficient diet, 141
  feeding frequency of, 100
  feeding pattern in hyperphagic, 98
  food reinforcement in rehabilitated, 101-102
  germfree
    characteristics of, 146-155
    composition of semisynthetic diet for, 143-146
    contamination among, 145-146
    effect of monocontaminations in single vitamin-K-deficient, 147-148, 149
    elimination of cholic acid in conventional, 152, 153
    enlarged cecum in, 148-149, 150, 151-152
    epethelial cells of intestine of, 150
    frequency of deficiency symptoms in, and controls on vitamin-K-deficient diet, 146
    longer lifespan of, 159
    mortality of, on vitamin-K-deficient diet, 146
    mucin in feces and contents of large intestines of, 151
    normal intestinal flora in, and reduction of enlarged cecum, 149, 151
    prothrombin values in, with vitamin-K-deficiency, 146-148
    reduced motility and sensitivity to biologically active compounds in, 150
    serum-cholesterol values in, and control, 153, 154
    tryptic activity in feces of, 151
    urobilins in feces from, and conventional, 152
  input and output of nitrogen in adult, 42-43
  lesions, and emotional behavior in, 102-103
  lithium toxic in, 73
  as meal eaters, 100, 115
  as regulator of nutrients in absence of taste and smell, 114-115
  resistance to toxicity of gold thioglucose in, 102, 103
  selection of food in, 115
  soil as source of endosymbionts in, 154
  urobilins in feces from exgermfree, contaminated with clostridium, 152, 153

Recycling system, in closed ecology, 71-74
Recyclostat, to produce algae, 191, 192
Red-cell production, low atmospheric pressure and changes in, 39-40
Regenerable solid adsorbent system, for CO_2 separation, 167-168
Regenerable solid adsorbents, defined, 167
Regenerative algal systems, for space flight, 181-188
Regenerative system
 chemical, 160, 161
 for Martian mission, 160-161
 reexamination of, 160-203
 weight of materials and, 204, 205-206
Reward, and feeding, 104
Rhythm, establishment of, by entraining, 108-109
Ristellae, defined, 125

Satiety
 and appetite, 92-118
 and hunger, 97
Scavengers, free radical, and antioxidants, 80, 84-85
Sea Lab, experiments in, 110
Selenium
 biological essentiality of, 56
 and deficiency disease, 61-62
 derivatives of, 62-63
 as dietary agent, 61-62
 organic chemistry of, 62
Semipermeable membranes
 concept of, for CO_2 separation, 169-170
 defined, 169
Serum cholesterol, and carbohydrates and diets, 31-32
Shielding, from radiation, 77
Sitodrepa panicea L., effect of symbiont removal in, 120
Sleep cycle, 111
Sleep-wakefulness cycle, in astronauts, 108
Smog, peroxyacetyl nitrate in, 77
Soil, as source of endosymbionts in rats, 134
Solar energy systems, 162-164
Solar flares, radiation from, 75
Solid absorbents, regenerable, for space flight, 167
Space, and unconventional or synthesized food, 28-29
Space capsule
 designing of, 81
 exposure to radiation in, 75
 temperatures, 164-165
Spacecraft
 cabin temperature in, 88-90
 germfree, 157
 overheating in, 89
 oxygen pressure within tissues in, 82
 reduction of temperature in, 88-89
Space flight
 bioregenerative algal systems for, 180-188
 calorie intake and expenditure of, in, 207-210
 chemical synthesis of food for, 176-179
 closed ecology for, 116
 control of CO_2 in, 166-176
 control of gaseous contaminants in, 137-138
 establishing cycles in, 112, 113
 exposure to radiation during, 75
 food forms for, 210-213
 four phases of, 161-176 *passim*
 man and bacterial flora on, 224
 nutrient requirements for, 206-210
 Phase I, 161
  chemical power, 162, 163
  lithium hydroxide for CO_2 control, 166-167
  oxygen supply, 162
 Phase II, 161
  CO_2 control in, 171
  regeneration system, 167
 Phase III, 162
  CO_2 control in, 171
  chemically regenerable systems, 171-176
  water supply for, 162-163
 Phase IV, 162
 Phases I–II, water supply for, 162-163
 Phases I–III, food and wastes in, 163
 Phases I–IV, vehicle systems in, 164
 Phases II–IV
  oxygen supply for, 162-163
  solar or nuclear energy for, 162, 163-164, 165
 Phases III–IV, bioregenerative systems in, 163

Phases III–IV—Continued
power sources, 162
regenerative algal systems for, 181-188
systems for phases of, 166-176 *passim*
vital aspects of life support for, 162-163
vitamin requirements in, 90-91
waste "storage," 166
weight of food for, 116
Space missions, essential characteristics of, 161
Sports, optimal diets for, 50-51
Staphylococcus aureus
and enterocolitis, 129
in nose, 129
overgrowth, 156
in stools, 129
Starving, versus fasting, 106
Stress, and food, 106-107
Submariners, food preferences of, 93-94
Sulhydryl compounds, as protections from radiation, 77
Sweating, heat-induced, 41
Symbiosis, 119-121

Taste, and odor, 114-115
Temperature
for bioregenerative systems, 179
cabin, in spacecraft, 88-90
effect of, on food in spacecraft, 88-90
and intake of food, 101
reduction of, in spacecraft, 88-89
Thirst, and dehydration, 21
Thyroid, desiccated, in diets, 70
Tolerance, 54
Toxicity, of astronauts to organisms, 221
Trace analysis, 64
Trace elements
behavior of, 59
biological tolerances for, 63
competition of, 60
controlled environment for deficiencies of, 65-71
discovery of requirements of, 55
essential, 55-56, 65
unidentified, 64-65
for mammalian organism, 69
monitoring of, in space, 64
prooxidative effects of, 87-88
toxicity and tolerance in, 63-64
Trace-element deficiency, 56, 66-68
Trace-element-free system, 56
Trace-element requirements, selectivity and specificity of, in nutrition, 59
Trace metals
antagonistic properties of, 60-61
toxic levels of, in recycled systems, 72
Transferrin, chromium transported by, 58

Urine
analysis of, after diet trials, 30-31
lack of specimens from flights, 18
water reclaimed from, 72-73

Van Allen belt, radiation in, 75
Veillonelle alcalescens, forms propionic acid, 125
Villi, bacterial contamination of mucosal, 140
Vitamin-A deficiency, 90-91
Vitamins, and variation in requirements in space flight, 90-91

Waste
disposal of, 221
as problem on space flights, 116, 118
Watch cycle, 112-113
Water
balance of, in astronauts, 88
reclaimed from urine, 72-73
recycling of, 116, 185
on space flights, 19-20
Weight, of materials, and regenerative systems, 204, 205-206

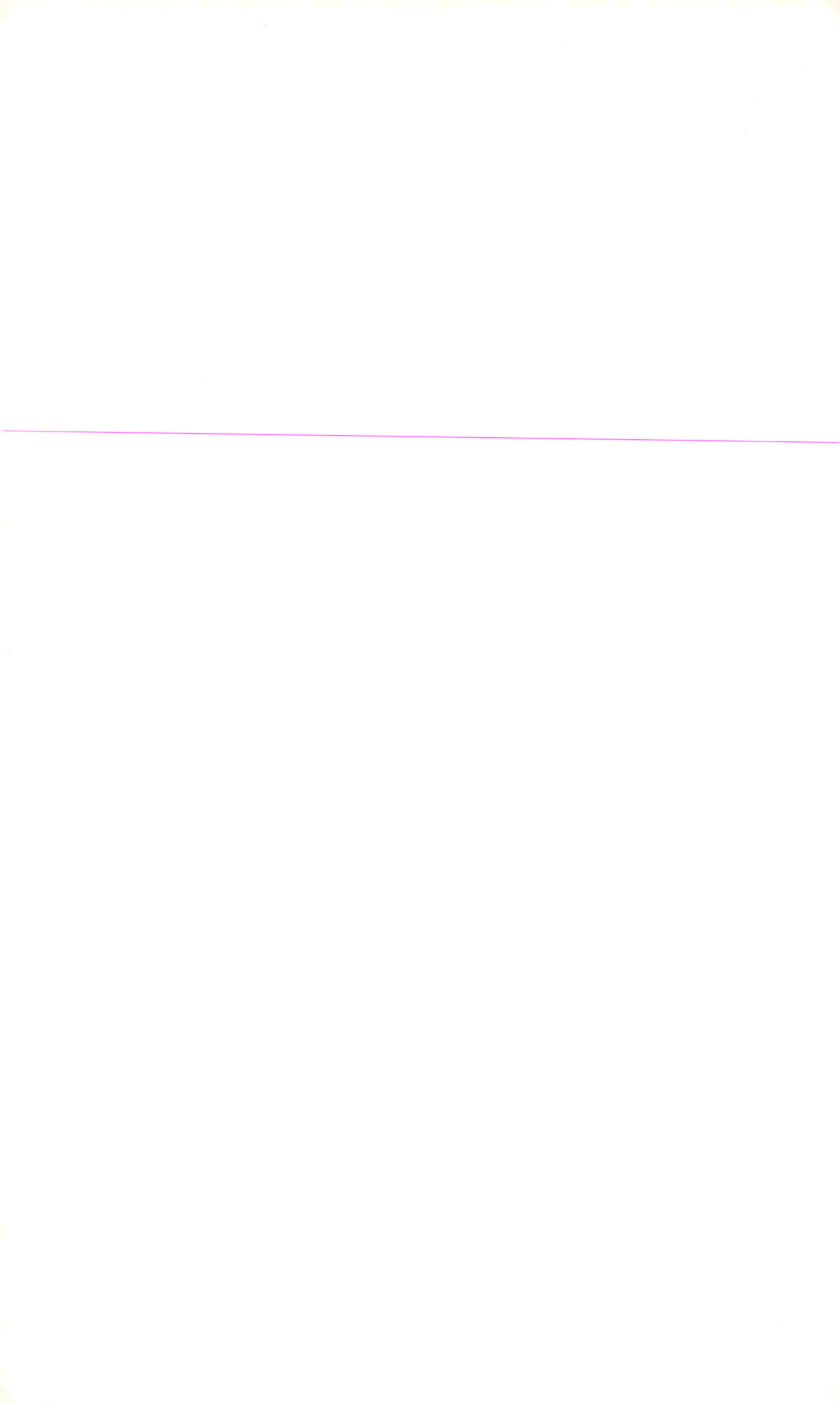

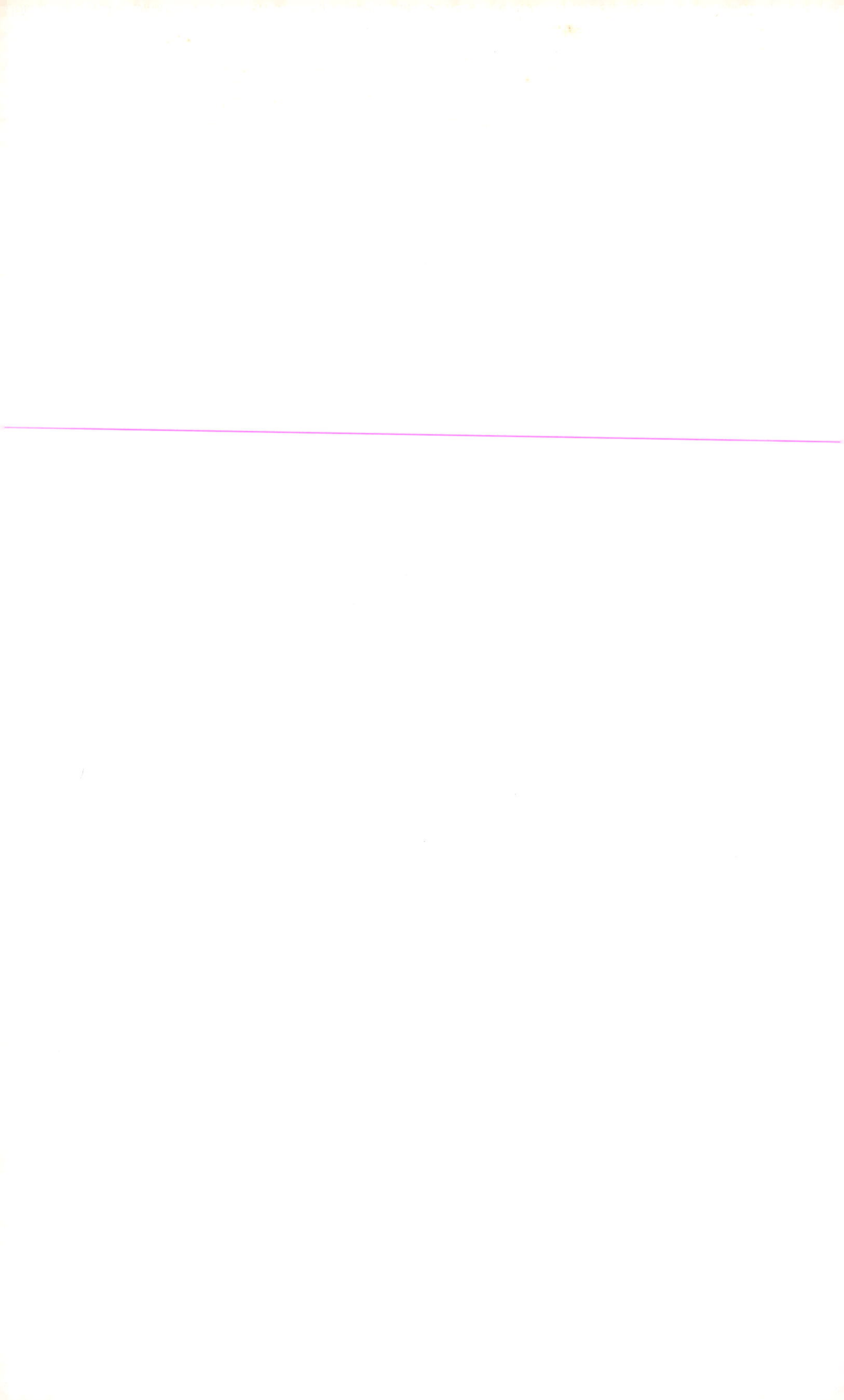

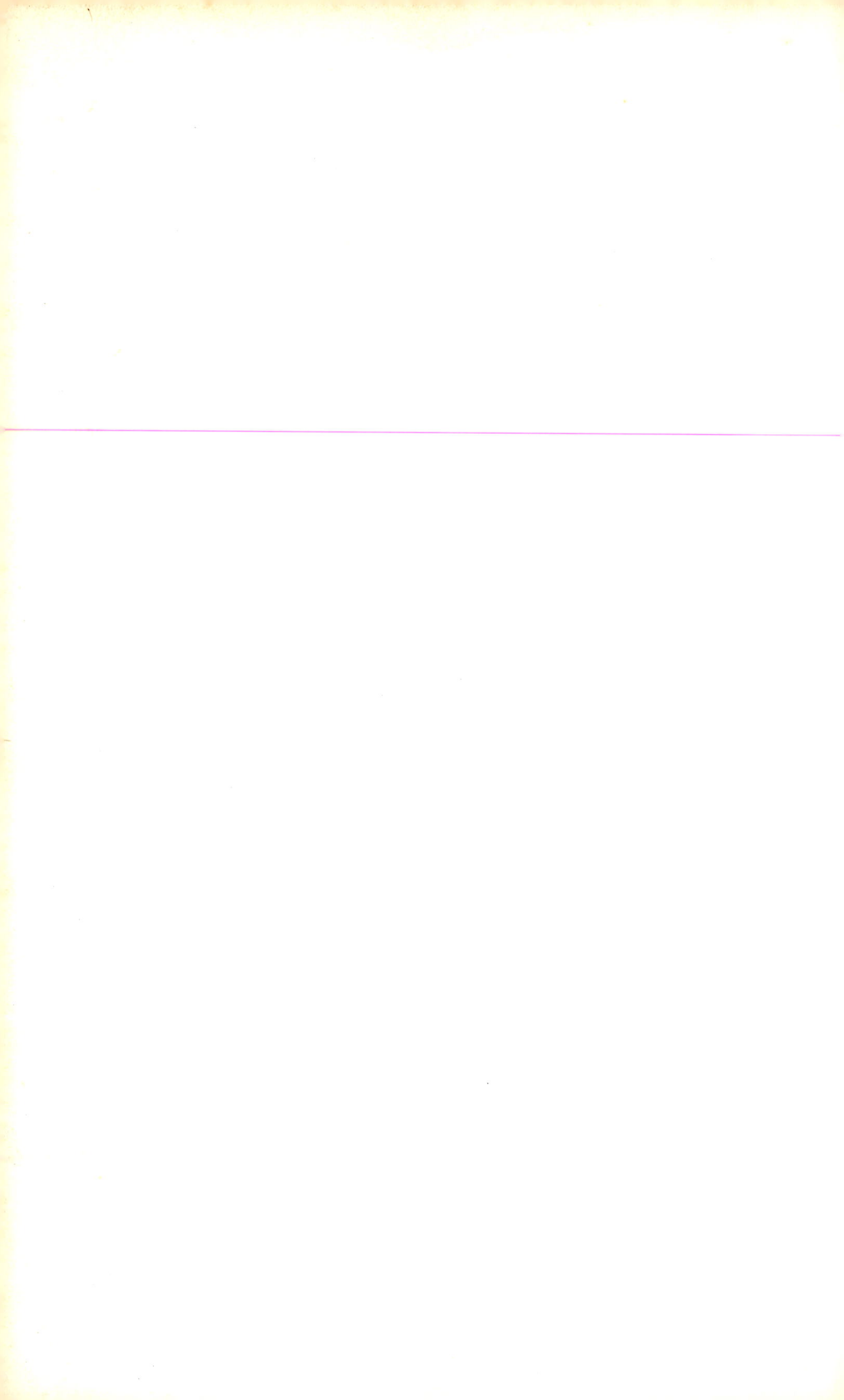